Pra

"A shocking scientific dete[...] wn.
Jason Dearen's skill at unrav[...] .ption
is matched only by his storytelling chops."

—Seth Mnookin, *New York Times*–bestselling author of *The Panic Virus:*
A True Story of Medicine, Science, and Fear

"Dearen unfolds his story like the murder mystery it sadly is. *Kill Shot*
also is a postmortem on a medical system gone alarmingly astray, told
by a writer who is as skilled at storytelling as fact-gathering, and whose
journalism helped expose the perpetrators."

—Larry Tye, *New York Times*–bestselling author of *Demagogue:*
The Life and Long Shadow of Senator Joe McCarthy

"A shocking, fascinating, edge-of-your-seat thrill ride, *Kill Shot* exposes
the dark underbelly of American medicine. It's a must-read for anyone
interested in the future of health care."

—Matt McCarthy, MD, author of *Superbugs: The Race to Stop an Epidemic*

"Ace investigative reporting, meticulous science writing, and Agatha
Christie suspense power—Jason Dearen's *Kill Shot*, a potent exposé on
the deadly consequences of greed and lax oversight in the drug industry.
Dearen's in-depth tale of how fungal meningitis spread from one
compounding pharmacy to kill and maim Americans in multiple states
is an indictment of self-regulation and a call to action to protect patients
from even greater harm."

—Cynthia Barnett, author of *Rain: A Natural and Cultural History*

KILL
SHOT

A Shadow Industry, a Deadly Disease

JASON DEAREN

AVERY | AN IMPRINT OF PENGUIN RANDOM HOUSE | NEW YORK

AVERY

an imprint of Penguin Random House LLC
penguinrandomhouse.com

First trade paperback edition 2022

ISBN (hardcover) 9780593085783
ISBN (e-book) 9780593085790
ISBN (trade paperback) 9780593421352

Printed in the United States of America

1st Printing

Book design by Lorie Pagnozzi

For Steph
And for my mother,
Della Betzina (1952–1992)

_____

CONTENTS

AUTHOR'S NOTE

This is a true story. The material in this book comes from interviews with more than a hundred and fifty sources, shoe-leather reporting in eight different states and Washington, D.C., and tens of thousands of pages of public documents.

All of the scenes included here were reconstructed using a wide range of sources: videos, photographs, transcripts, emails, personal handwritten notes, in-person and telephone interviews, U.S. Food and Drug Administration inspection reports and emails, and visits to the places where the scenes occurred.

Most of the people who appear in this book were interviewed in person, and many shared documents including medical records, calendars, and emails that helped me piece together their stories. For those who declined to be interviewed, I used transcripts of their testimony in multiple federal criminal trials and before the grand jury, as well as documents produced as evidence, which are public records. Most quotes were transcribed from videos, emails, trial transcripts, and inspection or investigative reports. When that wasn't possible I relied on interviews with people involved to reconstruct the conversation.

More details on the sourcing of each of the book's scenes can be found in the notes section.

During the nearly three years I spent reporting this book, I gave everyone multiple opportunities to participate through interviews or written questions and answers. I made multiple requests for interviews with Barry Cadden and Glenn Chin by letter and contact with their attorneys. They both declined.

PROLOGUE

ALBANY, KENTUCKY

The gravedigger arrived just after sundown, the night already full of the trills of crickets and katydids. He headed to the top of the cemetery's hill and pushed his shovel into the earth quietly, chunking out the grass and weeds on top before hitting soil. He was careful not to attract the attention of the residents of the small homes adjoining the site or of those in cars traveling along North Cross Street, the town's nearby thoroughfare.

The deceased was a judge, Eddie Lovelace, and his funeral a few weeks earlier had lasted hours, with what seemed like the entire 2,000-person town in attendance. State troopers, farmers in bibbed overalls and boots, even a man the judge had sent to jail twice came to pay their respects.

Two weeks before his death, the judge had still been presiding over criminal cases in the Colonial-style courthouse a few blocks from his house. The seventy-eight-year-old still walked three miles every morning—the same route down to the Talbott Funeral Home, then over to the Clinton County Hospital. Eleven days before his funeral he had collapsed after stepping off his porch to retrieve the

Lexington Herald-Leader from the mailbox. He had staggered to his feet and made it back to his kitchen, paper in hand, calling to his wife, Joyce, and waking her up. She immediately noticed that his face looked different. "My legs just aren't working," he'd said. She hurried to call her daughter, Karen, a nurse who lived down the street.

The next day, as Lovelace lay in a hospital room at Vanderbilt University Medical Center, a neurologist confirmed that he'd had an atypical stroke, in an unusual part of the brain.

A few days later, his speech had become too garbled to understand. Then he lost his ability to breathe or move his extremities. When his granddaughter asked for a thumbs-up, he managed only a weak response. Doctors still saw brain activity—he was in there—but he was "locked in."

The judge died a week after arriving at Vanderbilt. The cause of death was listed as unknown, and he was buried a few blocks from his small house on Lovelace Street, which had been named in his honor.

L ess than a month later, the gravedigger scooped out a couple of feet of dirt before his blade reached the top of Lovelace's cement vault. The weight of the earth above it had already created a tight seal, but a few swings from a sledgehammer cracked the vault open, interrupting the quiet.

The next morning, a hearse drove three hours north to Louisville, where the body was unloaded and taken into a low-slung mortuary building. The exhumed corpse was eased onto a stainless-steel table. The judge was still dressed in his robes, a gavel in his right hand. A key to the front door of his house was in his pocket, where he always kept it.

The medical examiner cut open the remains and studied each major organ. Multiple areas of the judge's brain showed evidence of hemorrhaging. As the pathologist reached the top of the spine, he noticed a growth covering the base of the brain stem—a microorganism, a translucent jellylike mold.

This was unheard of: a deadly mold blooming in the central nervous system of an otherwise healthy person. The medical examiner scraped out a sample and placed it in a sterile container for the lab.

After the judge's swift death, his family and community had buried him and started grieving. That was before they learned of the U.S. government's murder investigation. The expanding list of casualties. The injections. The source.

The judge had been buried before many others, but now his body and the microbe that had colonized his brain were evidence.

KILL
SHOT

CHAPTER 1

PATIENT ZERO

TWO MONTHS EARLIER

SMYRNA, TENNESSEE

Thomas Rybinski stood on his boat and looked out over the sparkling lake, the humidity enveloping him like a soggy blanket. It was a Saturday in August 2012, and he and his wife, Collette, had met two other couples for a weekend boating trip. The weather was ideal: light winds, the water surface glassy. The engine hummed as Rybinski piloted the bass boat into their favorite cove, where they anchored and grilled dinner. It was the perfect antidote to a day that had started strangely.

Rybinski had been unsteady since breakfast. From dawn to dusk, the fifty-five-year-old father of three was usually a blur of action. But when he had swung his legs out of bed that morning, he could move only gingerly, and he felt chills and nausea. His head hurt, and as he drank his morning cup of coffee he rubbed his hand over his head to try and quiet the banging inside. He thought it was probably a sinus headache. Still, Captain Tom, as his friends referred to him, kept his boating date. Out on the water he'd started to feel better, but the headache still bothered him; the next day they cut their trip short and went home.

On Monday, Rybinski felt well enough to work. For thirty-five years he'd been at General Motors, most recently as an auto designer. He was popular at GM and still youthful in middle age, although after long rides on his Harley his lower back flared up because of a bulging disk. Rybinski did not like to miss work—he loved cars, loved talking about them—and he got steroid injections that made the pain tolerable for months at a time.

By the end of the week Rybinski's mind was foggy and he walked with a slump. He told Collette, "I feel like the inside of my head is going to explode." Collette thought he might have the flu. On August 26, about a week after the boating trip, he went to Vanderbilt University Medical Center, a dense collection of Lego-like buildings in the heart of Nashville. His symptoms were consistent with meningitis, an infection some physicians describe as a swollen central nervous system. It's marked by inflammation of the meninges, the membranes that protect the spinal cord and brain stem. But Rybinski was not at high risk for meningitis. He had not been around a large group of people who could transfer bacteria, nor had he recently had surgery. His doctor looked elsewhere for an explanation. Rybinski had gone hiking in Colorado about a month earlier; perhaps a tick bite had introduced a pathogen? He was tested for Rocky Mountain spotted fever, a tick-borne bacterial disease with symptoms similar to meningitis. Such a diagnosis, while serious, was also possibly good news: most serious bacterial infections can be treated with antibacterial drugs. Still, Rybinski's doctors could not be sure until they tested his spinal fluid.

They checked him in to the hospital and gave him antibiotics and drugs to reduce the swelling. To everyone's relief, Rybinski regained his sharpness. After five days, they installed a catheter in his arm so he could administer the medications to himself, and he went home.

A few days later the headaches were back. Since being discharged, Rybinski had had a couple of good days, when he seemed like his old self. But he was declining quickly, and Collette had seen enough. She called in to work, grabbed his medications, and drove them to the closest emergency room to avoid the heavily trafficked twenty-four-mile trip to Vanderbilt. By the time they arrived, he was speaking gibberish. The doctor ordered an ambulance to take him back to Vanderbilt. There, in intensive care, Rybinski moved in and out of consciousness. One of the times he came to, he could not remember their wedding. It broke Collette's heart.

VANDERBILT UNIVERSITY MEDICAL CENTER

Dr. April Pettit walked down the hushed, fluorescent-lit hallway in Vanderbilt's critical care unit, the beeping of machines and the murmur of nurses greeting her as she started her shift. Just a year earlier, she had finished her fellowship and been hired by Vanderbilt as an attending physician. The thirty-four-year-old Pettit had a degree in public health and expertise in infectious disease. But she had little experience with cases of meningitis like the one in the patient she'd just inherited. She scanned his paperwork. Thomas Rybinski was a man in his fifties who had been healthy except for the back pain he felt when he rode his motorcycle. He was deteriorating quickly from meningitis of an unknown origin. To complicate matters, he could speak but was not making sense, so she had to rely on his medical records and his previous interviews with her colleagues for clues.

Pettit studied Rybinski's medical history and charts. Her first task was to build a differential diagnosis, a list of possible causes of his meningitis and stroke, ranked from the most likely to the least.

From there, she would move from the top of the list to the bottom, methodically ruling out potential causes one at a time. Bacterial meningitis was still the odds-on favorite, but he had not responded to antibiotics, and they had started him on an antifungal, too, just in case. There were other meningitis-causing microbes she needed to cross off the list, like viruses. So far all the labs were coming back negative, including a battery of tests of Rybinski's spinal fluid. She was still waiting for the results of a fungal culture, even though fungal meningitis had almost never been diagnosed in previously healthy people like Rybinski. Fungi usually have no clear pathway to a human spinal column. In fact, the lab at Vanderbilt had not grown a fungus in a spinal fluid sample for nearly thirty years. But Rybinski was short on time. At the very least, a negative culture would allow Pettit to cross fungus off her differential diagnosis.

Across the street, inside a sterile room the size of a walk-in refrigerator, the lab tech had put three samples of Rybinski's spinal fluid into separate vials. One held a sugary solution called Sabouraud agar, another used a form of mucus, and another was a crimson concoction of blood and brain matter. (The tech had performed these cultures for decades, but that last one still grossed her out.) Typically, if the fluid stays clear after a week or two, it's considered free of microbes. But some fungi could take weeks to show up, and hospital officials decided to monitor the culture until the process had run its course. While this was sound medical practice, it was also a problem: Rybinski's condition continued to worsen.

Six days after Rybinski was readmitted, his face was drooping on the right side, a sign of an intensifying stroke. A CT scan of his head revealed excess fluid around the brain. The doctors also found blocked oxygen-providing arteries in the back of his head.

In Rybinski's scans, reproduced later in *The New England Journal of Medicine*, the ghostly image of his brain is clearly *wrong*: tidy folds of tissue are interrupted by what looks like an off-white cluster in the center. Even to a layperson, it is obvious that this mass should not be there. Notes attached to the scan identified the anomaly as a pool of blood that collected near where the brain and spine meet. Similarly, the arteries that fed his brain were weakened by aneurysms, which had burst and bled into surrounding areas. These were the obvious ravages of an invasive species adapting to an unfamiliar ecosystem: Rybinski's central nervous system. There it had grown and multiplied, interrupting the flow of blood to his brain. This caused a stroke. What the images did not explain was exactly what was causing this or why.

The next day, in a refrigerator behind a door marked BIOHAZARD, one of Rybinski's cultures started changing. Where there had been clear spinal fluid, there was now a fuzzy mound of blue-green—the microbe up close. The technician was shocked. She needed to report the results immediately.

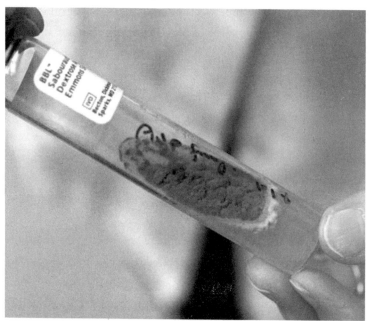

A culture of the fungus *Aspergillus fumigatus* grown at Vanderbilt University Medical Center in Nashville, Tennessee, during the fungal meningitis outbreak in October 2012. *(Courtesy of Shelley Mays/USA Today Network)*

Pettit stood with her medical fellow in Rybinski's cramped room in the intensive care unit (ICU), the only sounds coming from his softly beeping monitor. Collette was sitting in a chair near her husband's bed when the fellow's pager lit up. It was the lab. The medical fellow left the room to check in, and returned with Rybinski's results promptly. Pettit asked that the results be shared with Collette. This was an excruciating part of the job. The fellow said that Rybinski's culture had grown a fungus. Pettit felt relieved at a diagnosis, but also confused by it. She had heard of mold meningitis in organ transplant and HIV patients, whose immune systems were compromised by their conditions. She knew that mold could also cause infections in people with open wounds or cuts, but rarely meningitis. Rybinski simply did not fit any profile she had seen or read.

Pettit took a moment to collect her thoughts. She explained that a fungus was the likely cause of his sickness. She had no idea how it had gotten into him, but that didn't matter at the moment. It was attacking with impunity, and suddenly she had a tantalizing clue. She could now focus Rybinski's treatment with antifungal drugs to fight the infection. Within days, some blood tests showed improvement. But his brain function continued to deteriorate. He was in and out of a coma. CT scans showed heavy bleeding in the rear of his brain, and the volume of fluid there had also increased.

Back in her office, Pettit scoured the medical literature for any similar cases. Her staff waded through the Internet for something, anything, that would guide them. There was one article that perhaps contained a clue. After the 2004 tsunami that devastated Southeast Asia and killed 225,000 people, there had been a cluster of fungal meningitis cases at a clinic in Indonesia. Investigators traced the source to medical supplies used to administer epidurals to women during childbirth. The equipment had been stored in a humid, flooded warehouse. Investigators later reported that sealed packages holding needles used for the epidurals were covered in fungus, but desperate doctors had used them on six women anyway.

Pettit moved quickly. Among the first items she noted on Rybinski's paperwork was that he had received epidural steroid injections the previous summer at the St. Thomas Outpatient Neurosurgical Center across town. There was enough of a parallel with the Indonesia cases that Pettit thought she should report it to Tennessee's state health officials. Rybinski's doctor at St. Thomas performed fifteen to twenty epidural injections a day, and the clinic averaged 160 each week. It was a lucrative business that paid doctors 60 percent of the revenue from each patient, and there were always people in pain. She typed up the case details quickly into an email.

Unbeknownst to her, another St. Thomas clinic patient had been admitted into Vanderbilt's ICU, just down the hall from Rybinski: Judge Eddie Lovelace. Because the judge's stroke so swiftly took away his ability to communicate, his doctors didn't know about his headaches, nausea, or the other signs of meningitis. They had no reason to order a spinal tap or test for a microbial invader.

DAY 1, SEPTEMBER 18, 2012: ONE CASE

TENNESSEE DEPARTMENT OF HEALTH, NASHVILLE
Pettit's email set off alarm bells in Dr. Marion Kainer's head.

"We have a case of a 55yo immunocompetent man with *Aspergillus fumigatus* meningitis," Pettit wrote, using the scientific name for the common fungal species identified by Vanderbilt's lab. "He had been receiving lumbar epidural steroid injections at an outside facility which is the only explanation we can find to explain this. He also has an L4–L5 1cm epidural abscess which supports this theory. I wanted to inform you of this in case you feel that an investigation is warranted."

Kainer, one of the state's chief medical detectives, called Pettit immediately. "Tell me everything from the beginning," she said.

The Tennessee Department of Health operates within a network of state and federal agencies that employ epidemiologists like Kainer—doctors responsible for tracking and finding the cause of disease outbreaks. In the case of a sexually transmitted disease like HIV, public health officials study how it has been transmitted and to whom, and then find ways to reduce exposure and death. The stakes are always high when Kainer launches an investigation. Each day that passes without answers means illness can spread.

A native Australian who speaks with a caffeinated intensity, Kainer had studied brain science before she refocused on epidemiology, motivated by a devastating epidemic at a hospital in Melbourne that killed one of her patients. The cause was a drug-resistant infection plaguing hospitals worldwide called methicillin-resistant *Staphylococcus aureus*, or MRSA. An especially robust bacterium with a thick cell wall, MRSA can fend off the antibacterial agents used in cleaning products, making it hard to eradicate. As a clinician, Kainer knew how to research diseases and prescribe treatments. The loss of her patient to MRSA had rocked her confidence. When it came to investigating the cause of a disease—epidemiology—Australia in the early 1990s was far behind the United States.

She applied to the Epidemic Intelligence Service (EIS) at the U.S. Centers for Disease Control and Prevention (CDC) in Atlanta. The two-year program is a disease detective's West Point. The agency plays a part in fighting everything from annual flu outbreaks to Ebola. Since finishing her training at the CDC, Kainer had made a name for herself as an aggressive investigator.

Now Tom Rybinski's file was in front of her. It was only one person, not even a cluster of cases, but the disease was rare and unexplained. How would the fungus infecting his central nervous system have gotten there? Something as simple as a leaky air conditioner or ice machine could cause a mold problem at a pain clinic or hospital, and Rybinski had been in both in the past eight weeks. In particular, construction work—a regular occurrence at most big-city medical centers—could spread fungal spores by opening up walls. But staff at Vanderbilt were checking for any mold growths in their facilities and so far had found nothing troubling. Kainer also called the St. Thomas pain clinic, where the manager was on vacation. Kainer was concerned, but one case was not a full-on emergency. So she waited.

Three days later, Kainer got a call back from the clinic manager. There had been no construction and no mold problems at the St. Thomas clinic, either. But there was troubling news: two other patients had called in reporting dizziness, a stiff neck, and other meningitis-like symptoms.

THE U.S. CENTERS FOR DISEASE CONTROL AND PREVENTION, ATLANTA

Dr. Benjamin Park had already seen a lot in his decade at the CDC—patients blinded by fungal infections due to tainted contact lens solution, children dying from the flu, and dozens of nurses sickened during the global outbreak of the coronavirus SARS-CoV. Each case represented a vexing life-threatening puzzle, and Park had become a seasoned investigator.

A slender and boyish man who was just turning forty, he had the calm manner of someone who'd witnessed his share of death up close. His office overlooked the CDC's campus, a labyrinthine collection of modern buildings with green-tinted windows, connected by underground tunnels. CDC scientists develop everything from antidotes for chemical weapons like anthrax to experimental treatments for rare infections that appear without warning. This agency is designed to be the brain of the nation's response to disease epidemics.

Park studied the world through the lens of a microscope and had found his calling as a specialist investigating diseases caused by molds and other fungi. He had always loved a good detective story, but his epidemiology courses in medical school had not captured his imagination and he'd been on a path to become a clinician. That changed one day during his rounds as a resident in Ann Arbor. The school invited a speaker from the Epidemic Intelligence Service to convince doctors to join the CDC's detective corps. Listening to the talk, Park envisioned a way to merge his medical training and his love of mathematics to solve high-stakes mysteries. Plus, the corps offered a concentration in medical mycology, the study of human fungal pathogens and a vital area of public health. As a clinician, he'd seen fungal infections ravage people, especially those weakened by illness like cancer. Once a fungus invaded, these at-risk patients often died, because there are far fewer drugs available to fight fungal diseases; antifungal medications are hard to develop. Perhaps epidemiology would give him the tools to help more than the one patient at a time.

It was a quiet Thursday when Kainer's email popped into his in-box. Tennessee was requesting help from the CDC, and Kainer wanted to know if they had heard of any fungal meningitis cases in the United States. Park had not, but a brain-altering fungus could be a serious public health concern.

At the moment, Kainer had only one confirmed fungal meningitis patient, Rybinski, but a couple of others had cropped up at the same clinic. These new cases had arrived at St. Thomas Hospital—which was affiliated with the neurosurgical clinic—with signs of meningitis. Kainer already recognized that the situation warranted a more aggressive investigation, and Park agreed.

On the same day that Eddie Lovelace's granddaughter sang at his funeral at Albany First Baptist, Kainer sent out a health alert in Tennessee for all clinics and hospitals to report any patients who had meningitis-like symptoms following an epidural injection. Since the alert went out, her phone had been ringing nonstop. Within hours, she'd received reports of four more possible cases from doctors in Nashville. Two of the cases had experienced stroke in the same part of the brain as Rybinski and had deteriorated quickly.

Confirming these new cases would be tricky. The patients were all having cerebrospinal fluid removed for a fungal culture, but the results could take weeks, and they did not have the luxury of time. If this was the same disease that Rybinski had, these patients could die in the weeks before a culture turned positive.

This was an ominous sign. If the number of cases spiked quickly, a time lag in diagnoses would be a problem for doctors in Tennessee who wanted to start to preventatively prescribe antifungal medications before a positive lab result. The drugs were expensive. One of the main antifungals they wanted to prescribe retailed for $2,000 per dose, and was in short supply. Without a diagnosis code, insurance companies would not cover them. The physicians had two bad choices: roll the dice on a pricey drug, or wait for results that could take more than a week and hope for the best.

In Atlanta, Park began digging around for similar previous cases. He found the same article that Pettit had read about the infected epidurals in Indonesia. But this didn't help with the real quandary. While Rybinski had tested positive for a fungus, none of the handful of other spinal fluid samples had yielded anything similar. Also, nothing as yet had been found at the clinic to account for a mold outbreak.

As Park worked methodically on the investigation, he also felt a growing dread; there were signs that this case might worsen, fast. They'd already ruled out their most promising hypothesis. The first patients had all been treated by only one person, Dr. John Culclasure. But the seventh to come forward had been injected by another St. Thomas doctor. If these cases were connected, this new variable would rule out a problem specific to Culclasure's procedure. But there was some good news, relatively speaking. All of the patients were still affiliated with just one place, the St. Thomas pain clinic. Whatever was happening, it appeared that the answers might lie inside the pain clinic's walls.

Kainer was looking at seven suspected fungal meningitis cases from the St. Thomas clinic, which had voluntarily closed down and sequestered all of its medical supplies. But only one spinal fluid culture had come back positive. She could not wait for more test results. Kainer needed records for everyone who had been treated there in the past few months: their ages, their allergies, the dates and number of injections they'd received. The information would help her calculate which patients were most at risk and where any new infections could occur. But the clinic's computers were incompatible with the state's and the patient files would not download. Kainer improvised, sending her staffers to manually transcribe each chart. The handwritten data was faxed across town to the health department office, where another employee began building a database.

As her staff collected patient data, Kainer began to pursue the infection's source. At the top of her list was a facility that had made steroids for the back-pain injections. The New England Compounding Center.

CHAPTER 2

THE FERRARI OF COMPOUNDERS

FRAMINGHAM, MASSACHUSETTS

Barry Cadden leaned forward in his chair, angling for a view of his small audience over a stack of papers. A dozen members of his sales force had gathered in the conference room, notepads at the ready. "All right. Welcome, everybody. So as we know, we're being filmed today. No goofy questions like the last time, right?" he said. It was May 2012, and this was the third sales training video Cadden had shot in recent days. In the prior session, some sales representatives had asked questions about legally sensitive subjects that he wanted to avoid.

Cadden's receding hairline and downcast eyes gave him a look of tired resignation. But his hands sliced energetically through the air as he spoke. "We're pioneers," he said, explaining to those in the room the company's decade-long role as, he believed, Good Samaritan in the national drug market. The United States had regularly faced supply shortages of many common medications—70 in

2006 had grown to 210 by 2011. There were many reasons for the shortfalls, not the least of which was that Big Pharma, brand-name companies like GlaxoSmithKline, Pfizer Inc., Johnson & Johnson, or Bristol-Myers Squibb, sometimes abandoned manufacturing certain drugs after they lost their lucrative patent protections. Also, drug manufacturers relied increasingly on a global supply chain that was prone to disruption. Some 80 percent of the raw materials in the pharmaceuticals sold in the U.S. are imported from Europe, India, or China, and if a foreign company had a problem—armed conflicts, political upheaval, trade disputes, animal diseases, contamination during transport—the U.S. market felt it. Amid these supply interruptions, hospital pharmacists were under intense pressure to keep important drugs on the shelf, but many medications were made in-house without preservatives and had a short shelf life. This made in-house compounding an expensive balancing act. How could a hospital make enough drugs to meet patient demand, but not so much that they would spoil on the pharmacy shelf and have to be discarded? During these frequent breakdowns in the supply chain, the steroids, antibiotics, and eye-numbing agents used in common surgeries were impossible to source, but still needed.

While Big Pharma decided what medications to make, big-box retailers like Walmart took over the pharmacy market in many communities, driving corner drugstores out of business. But Walmart and many other large retail pharmacies did not compound many drugs, creating an opportunity for down-on-their-luck pharmacists. In stepped more nimble operations like the New England Compounding Center.

Federal law allowed compounding pharmacies to customize medicines for special-needs patients. If a child needed a lower dose of a commercially available drug, like a painkiller, or someone was allergic to a binding agent in their synthetic thyroid hormones, the patient's doctor wrote a prescription and a compounding pharmacist made it from "active pharmaceutical ingredients" (APIs), the chemical constituents of drugs, and excipients like fillers or bulking agents. For hundreds of years, this kind of work was a normal part of an apothecary/pharmacist's duties, and the practice was thus exempted from many federal drug safety regulations passed in the early twentieth century. By the 1980s, as mass-manufactured drugs under the purview of the U.S. Food and Drug Administration became dominant, the practice of compounding became a niche part of the business. Then, by the start of the 2000s, drug shortages made compounding a necessity once more.

It was a hero's narrative, and Cadden delivered it with a sincere confidence.

When Cadden's brothers-in-law, Gregory and Douglas Conigliaro, cofounded NECC in 1998, it was a family business, making small quantities of custom medications that no one else did. Because Douglas, an anesthesiologist, owned a pain-management practice in Florida, his ownership of NECC presented a legal conflict of interest. His siblings stepped in, and his wife, Carla, held a majority of the ownership in her name.

Douglas and Greg's sister, Lisa Conigliaro Cadden, and her husband, Barry, ran the day-to-day operations and held about a third of the company's shares. Even the company's location was a family affair. A sign in the parking lot advertised Conigliaro Block, Nationwide Foam, Inc., and Conigliaro Industries—all owned by Greg Conigliaro. Anyone arriving at the generic business park situated between a swamp and a pond in a neighborhood of plain clapboard houses would likely miss the pharmaceutical laboratory sandwiched between the concrete-block maker and a recycling center, their attention drawn instead to the hills of old mattresses and discarded furniture in the parking lot. Across the street, a sports pub that opened at 11:30 A.M. was a popular spot for employees.

In its first years, NECC had earned a few million dollars filling modest orders mostly to strip-mall pain clinics and doctors' offices, which could not afford to employ pharmacists to compound sterile drugs in-house. Federal law permitted compounding pharmacies to legally ship a percentage of their wares without a prescription— usually 5 percent, depending on the state—to other states for so-called office use, a small quantity that doctors could stock as an emergency supply. NECC had been relying on the office use exemption to compound an increasing quantity of popular medicines like the corticosteroid betamethasone, the heart-stopping cardioplegia drugs used by cardiac surgeons, and hundreds more without prescriptions. No one tracked exactly how many drugs NECC made or where they were shipping them; state and federal drug safety officials relied on compounding pharmacists like Cadden to honestly self-report. The practice was already lucrative, and Cadden saw room for exponential growth.

His first priority was building a sales force filled with what he called "killers"—sales reps like him who would go after hospital pharmacies aggressively.

Facing pressures from drug shortages and changing safety standards, many hospitals had started making so-called high-risk drugs in-house. These were the sterile drugs injected into people's hearts, backs, and eyes that require the highest level of aseptic technique to produce safely. ("We don't like the term *high risk* because it has negative connotations," Cadden said.) In 2007, the United States Pharmacopeia, the industry's standard-bearer since 1820, had begun to update their safety guidelines and present hospitals and surgery centers with a stark choice. Hospitals would have to invest in expensive sterile labs called clean rooms, as well as equipment and training. Or they could outsource the work to compounding pharmacies.

When the USP began to update its standards in 2007, Cadden

saw an opportunity. He had fourteen sales reps for the entire United States, only two of whom concentrated on hospitals, at a time when Big Pharma employed a hundred thousand. As he let go of existing employees, he hired new recruits whom he could remake in his own image, until finally the department had a cutthroat atmosphere.

Watching over the group was national sales director Rob Ronzio, whom Cadden had hired to help him grow the business. Ronzio, as everyone called him, had the stout build of a former hockey player and a pugilistic demeanor. If Cadden had a platonic ideal in mind of an NECC salesman, Ronzio was it. Ronzio had heard about the job opening from an old college hockey coach. For Cadden, himself a former athlete who prized intense competitors, it was kismet. His sales reps would need to be both smart enough to understand the complexity of the drug market and comfortable swimming in the uncertain waters that came with venturing into legal gray areas. Ronzio had no experience in pharmaceuticals, but he had an innate talent for selling. When Cadden told him that a sales rep should think like a hunter stalking his prey, they were speaking the same language.

With Ronzio, Cadden set out to nurture his sales force. These seminars were a way to do that. Reps could take the recordings with them as they traveled around the country. A natural performer, Cadden beamed when he got a laugh. "Does every compounding pharmacy out there do exactly what we do? Absolutely not. They don't have the same equipment, the same people, the same procedures," he said, his hands working the air. NECC had a different way of doing things that gave them an edge.

That edge was a willingness to exploit loopholes. Cadden alluded to just enough so the recruits would understand. The nation's laws on compounding had been designed with your basic corner retail pharmacy in mind, he explained, mixing small batches of drugs for individual patients based on a doctor's prescription. Big Pharma was still making most of the nation's medicines in factories subject to the U.S. Food and Drug Administration's safety guidelines and oversight, which included unannounced inspections. The FDA's Current Good Manufacturing Practices (CGMPs) were a complex tangle of rules meant to promote safety in the country's foods and medicines. Complying with even these minimum requirements meant years of slow, costly improvements.

When the demand for compounding began to increase in the nineties, Congress and the FDA scrambled to catch up. In 1997, Congress passed the Food and Drug Administration Modernization Act (FDAMA). Section 503A still exempted small-time low-risk compounding from standard drug approval requirements. It focused instead on the more egregious practices of large-volume compounding businesses. Pharmacies could no longer solicit doctor prescriptions, nor could they make drugs that were identical to a commercially available product, unless it was on the FDA's drug shortage list. A compounded medication had to be customized in some way. And pharmacies could neither market nor advertise their products. Doctors had to reach out to compounders when a patient needed a prescription, not vice versa. Under the FDAMA, if a compounding pharmacy did any of these things the FDA could shut them down, after a long process of warnings.

A group of compounding pharmacies sued, and in 2002 the Supreme Court weighed in on a key issue in the case. With a 5–4 split decision in *Thompson v. Western States Medical Center*, the ruling paved the way for compounding pharmacies to continue to market and advertise drugs. The ruling paralyzed the FDA's years-long efforts.

The agency was hamstrung. What little oversight was available was left to a patchwork of state pharmacy boards. Compounding pharmacies such as NECC were being regulated like the corner druggist—not Pfizer—and Cadden wanted to keep it that way.

Without the FDA looking over their shoulders, Cadden's pharmacists could do things differently. Most important, they could move fast, getting drugs to customers in days. In a reference to competing pharmacies that played by the rules, Cadden put it this way: "You got to feel as though you're selling Ferraris and they're selling Yugos," referring to the cheap, notoriously ramshackle subcompact.

The only wrinkle in his plan for total domination was demand. Hospitals need lots of drugs, but NECC was, technically, a pharmacy. Just like the corner drugstore, it needed one key piece of paper to legally make and dispense most medicines: a doctor's prescription. After all, if pharmacists are required to have a prescription for each medicine, they cannot mass-produce drugs, meaning they are justifiably exempt from the FDA's strict good manufacturing practices.

This requirement was also bad for profit. So Cadden found a way around it. Massachusetts required doctors to sign an individual prescription for each patient, which was sent directly from doctor to pharmacy via a phone line; email was considered too insecure. This was a time-consuming chore for doctors who needed thousands of doses of medicines. NECC created pre-printed order forms that could be faxed from a hospital and which could contain multiple orders, but required only one signature from a doctor's office. It was a work-around that was technically legal—the doctor's signature was on there. In the unlikely event that a state pharmacy inspector asked Cadden for prescription records for the tens of thousands of vials and syringes made by NECC, Cadden believed the faxed-in order sheets would satisfy the letter of the law, if not its spirit.

Still facing the camera, Cadden stopped speaking abruptly, leaned back, and grinned. He had learned that one of the most powerful tools in sales is fear. When it came to doctors, that might be the fear of making mistakes in mixing complicated medicines. The fear of killing someone. The fear of malpractice lawsuits. "This is how we help them. You give them more hours back. And the big dirty word is the liability issue," he said, his arms drawing circles, hands splayed like starfish.

Sending out drugs without patient prescriptions is illegal, and Cadden knew it. But the Massachusetts Board of Registration in Pharmacy was a chronically underfunded operation with only three investigators covering more than eleven hundred pharmacies. (Dozens of other states were in a similar boat.) It was responsible for overseeing forty-seven larger compounding pharmacies similar to NECC. One of the Massachusetts board's members, Sophia Pasedis, worked in co-owner Greg Conigliaro's office, helping manage another family-owned drug-compounding enterprise, Ameridose's, relationship with the board. In fact, Cadden claimed, the state oversight board was an extension of the pharmacy industry, meant to ward off federal scrutiny. As Cadden told his reps, "About seven years ago a handful of compounding pharmacies—a good-old-boy network—just said, 'Hey, we're going to make a little board thing and we'll go around, just you and me, and we'll go into your pharmacy and say, "You're good." And then you come into mine.' At that point in time, FDA was trying to grab compounding."

Not one of Massachusetts's three pharmacy inspectors was trained or qualified to inspect sterile rooms. And the FDA inspectors who were had to be invited in by the state board. "We're like a pimple on a flea's behind in pharmacies," he said, getting laughs. In the privacy of his conference room, he mimicked a scene from NECC's last state inspection. "They don't even know what they're looking at. They have no clue. They go around, like, 'Barry, this place looks great!'" he said with a snicker. "I give 'em a cup of coffee and out the door. That's what it is like!"

NECC revenues had spiked from $5 million in 2004, before the U.S. Pharmacopeia changed its safety standards, to $13.1 million in 2007, the year they changed. In 2011, the company took in $27.4 million, and as Cadden spoke in 2012, it was on track to earn nearly $50 million. NECC's drugs were cheaper than the brand names—they could pass on the savings of not having to comply with federal CGMPs—and were readily available. They would receive regular orders from 8,500 hospitals and their surgical clinics.

It was Cadden's job to keep it all on track. The sales team traveled constantly to drum up new business, attending trade shows and feting potential clients. He and his wife, Lisa, had recently built a $1.4 million, thirteen-room mansion and owned three other properties, including a waterfront weekend house in Rhode Island, held a $1.5 million trust, as well as luxury cars. The Conigliaros were also getting rich.

Cadden paused again. He'd been talking for a while and still had not explained how the "clean rooms" one floor below were going to handle the deluge of orders he expected them to bring in. Cadden had carefully separated the two parts of his business. The lab was behind a door that required a key card to enter, and the reps were never to communicate directly with the pharmacists. This gave them plausible deniability; they could not question Cadden's commitment to quality if they did not see evidence contradicting it. If a salesperson needed the lab to rush an order out or to change something, they had to go through Ronzio or Cadden's other consigliere, Sharon Carter, a stern, crisply dressed woman who oversaw order processing. Only the people who worked inside the clean room knew what was happening there. All anyone else needed to believe in faithfully and to communicate forcefully was one word: quality.

"The most important thing we do every day in the lab is produce quality—and understand that we do it. Understand that you should use that as part of your sales approach. Absolutely understand that we're not selling jelly beans. These are, you know, sterile products."

But achieving quality, sterility, is not easy. The colossal brand-name manufacturers like GlaxoSmithKline and Pfizer that make sterile drugs under FDA oversight are required to record each tiny step; when errors pop up, there is a diary of what went wrong. The system is onerous because it is designed to force profit-minded companies to protect the public health. Drugs made in these regulated factories often vary in strength and preparation. The FDA defines what minute levels of variance are considered safe, for example, between brand-name and generic drugs. It is an exacting process—one that compounding pharmacies like NECC are not required to follow.

Cadden's predilection to skirt safeguards had piqued the federal government's interest a decade earlier. In March 2002, the FDA suspected that a contaminated batch of the company's steroids had killed a man, William Koch, and sickened at least five other people with "meningitis-like symptoms." After a physician reported the problem to the FDA, inspectors visited NECC to evaluate Cadden's manufacturing processes. The FDA would file their concerns—which included letting a batch of steroids sit out for days with nothing but a piece of tinfoil covering the beaker—with the state board. The inspections also found that NECC kept no records. Cadden couldn't verify if his drugs met USP safety standards, and there was no way for NECC to respond to complaints or adverse events. One inspector noted in a report that Cadden was helpful on the first day, but after he spoke to a lawyer, everything changed: "From that point on it was essentially 'talk to my lawyer.'" The incident was settled quietly.

Later that year, Cadden made a batch of methylprednisolone acetate steroid that sickened at least two more people with meningitis-like symptoms, and the FDA returned for another round of inspections. This time the inspectors were more forceful, recommending to the Massachusetts oversight board that NECC be "prohibited from manufacturing until they can demonstrate ability to make product reproducibly [*sic*] and dependably." In response, Cadden wrote letters promising to make changes to his processes. He hired another pharmacist, bought equipment, and expanded the lab. The state launched a committee to update its regulations for compounding pharmacies, a recognition that the industry had grown beyond its control. The state appointed Cadden to serve on the committee.

In 2004, the Massachusetts board received a complaint from a surgical center in Rapid City, South Dakota, that NECC was selling drugs without legal prescriptions. The board investigated and sent NECC an advisory letter. The same day, it also looked into two other complaints about the company from pharmacists in Wisconsin and Iowa. Again, Cadden promised to clean up his act and the inquiries faded away.

Cadden did not mention any of these smudges on his record to his sales reps, of course. Instead, he encouraged them to counter any skepticism about NECC from doctors or hospital pharmacists by name-dropping: "Know in your area who our big clients are. The big names. I mean, use that stuff. Drop those names out there. They love that stuff." Indeed, the reps saw some well-known names on the roster, chief among them Massachusetts General Hospital in Boston. Association with the world-famous institution enhanced NECC's credibility. What Cadden didn't mention was that, after years of striking out with Mass General, NECC had finally landed the account with a tried-and-true tactic: payoffs. NECC and Ameridose started paying a pharmacy staffer, Claudio Pontoriero, $5,000 a month. In exchange, he steered orders for a variety of drugs

NECC's way, bringing in cash and cachet. The deal went unnoticed for five years, and earned Pontoriero more than $355,000.

Cadden's tone turned somber. He put his palms together as if in prayer. Hospitals had to trust that the reps were telling them the truth about the efforts NECC made to keep its drugs safe, and the reps had to trust Cadden. "We live and die with this place. I know if we don't produce quality this whole thing goes up in smoke . . . I know that," he said. The room was silent.

The most important factors, he continued, were all of the things that the sales team and clients never saw, like environmental monitoring for contaminants. NECC would indeed hire an employee to test the sterile rooms' air, work surfaces, and floors. She had no training in the discipline, but it allowed Cadden to boast in marketing materials about the company's commitment to safety.

Listening to Cadden felt like drinking from a fire hose, one sales rep at the seminar would say later. A pharmacy tech described a riveting display of self-confidence bordering on arrogance. But he had given them the practical and psychological tools they needed to sell to hospitals and surgery centers around the nation. NECC was competing with hundreds of other compounders, and even some hospitals' own pharmacies. But the competition was not as fast as NECC, Cadden said. If they used the script, they would be successful. "If you relay all the information that you should, as best you can, they're going to think about that. And that's a big part of your job—to relay that information to them. Okay? Go down that checklist."

NECC was making tens of millions of dollars annually. Cadden saw the potential for a great deal more.

NASHVILLE

Mario Giamei looked like a bouncer, but he carried himself with a gentle disposition. And in fact he had worked security at a Rhode

Island nightclub called the Station, which made national news in 2003 for a fire that killed a hundred people at a heavy metal concert. He worked with the Worcester County Sheriff's Department, at a cable company, and at a mortgage bank amid the financial crash of 2008. He knew Ronzio from previous business deals in Rhode Island. When Giamei showed up for his second interview at NECC two years earlier, Cadden told him he was looking for "hunters" who could close deals—salespeople who would make cold calls, knock on doors, and pressure potential customers into appointments. Like most of the sales reps, Giamei had no pharmaceutical experience, but he had a family and kids to support. Cadden recognized motivation when he saw it, and hired Giamei.

All recruits were given a booklet that listed NECC's products and described its state-of-the-art facilities. Cadden told them that customers should be assured that each drug was put through a battery of tests for contamination to ensure it was of the right strength and was free of contaminants. This was important; it set NECC apart.

Cadden also promised a tour of the clean rooms, but Giamei never managed to pin him down on this. Even though the pharmacists worked just a floor below him, whenever it came time to go downstairs, Cadden moved the date. Even so, Giamei was impressed with the procedures he had heard about to guarantee patient safety. He felt like he had a good product to sell and lots of bait with which to lure in clients.

The work wasn't always easy. The lowest performers on the sales staff were in constant jeopardy of being fired. Sometimes people were canned their first day on the job. The merciless atmosphere was simply the sign of a company on the rise, Ronzio would tell his sales reps. "This is what Barry wants for us."

The job could be exciting, too, with a sense of camaraderie. As a form of orientation, Ronzio took Giamei to Nashville to a conference with boxes of Cadden's brochure—a shabby-looking wire-bound booklet with clip-art graphics. The second page displayed a photo of a pharmacist in a hairnet, his face covered with a mask, and his arms in a sterile glove box, a sealed container in which drugs were mixed. What the booklet lacked in visual sophistication it made up for in sales psychology. Pharmacy directors and buyers at hospitals answered to the doctors, and wanted to know whether a medicine supplier complied with the sterile compounding rules of the U.S. Pharmacopeia. These handouts would disarm any skeptics.

Trade shows were a particularly rich feeding ground. In Nashville, Giamei was sent to an industry confab called the Tennessee Ambulatory Surgery Center Association Conference. Pain clinics and hospitals were heavily represented, so it was a perfect place to sell one of NECC's central products: pain-relieving steroids. Giamei set up the booth with a purplish blue banner reading: "Compounded by Pharmacists Extensively Trained in Aseptic Compounding." The word *aseptic* is holy writ to pharmacists and drug manufacturers, implying procedures like handwashing, equipment decontamination, and sterilization that are key to drug purity. Quality. Class.

At the conference Giamei met Debra Schamberg, the head nurse at a local pain clinic, the St. Thomas Outpatient Neurosurgical Center. The clinic was connected to a larger hospital in Nashville and was always busy. Its doctors did dozens of spinal injections each day, and Schamberg was on the hunt for a supplier of a steroid called methylprednisolone acetate. MPA, or methylpred, is a popular pain reliever for people with joint or back issues. There was a national shortage of the brand-name form of the drug, Depo-Medrol, and the clinic was having trouble getting their orders filled. NECC offered MPA on demand, and in a preservative-free form, which doctors preferred because it was less irritating for their patients.

As she chatted with Giamei, Schamberg took a flyer to share with her boss, Dr. John Culclasure. The flyer displayed a photo of NECC's main offering: a little brown bottle with a label reading *Steroids (Preservative-Free)*. Atop the list of medications NECC offered was its big moneymaker, methylprednisolone acetate, followed by bullet points about how the company was fully compliant with the USP sterile compounding guidelines. Schamberg left NECC's booth encouraged.

Back at the St. Thomas clinic, Culclasure glanced at the sheet. NECC's promise of reliable methylpred would be a bulwark against future shortages of Depo-Medrol and its generic counterparts. NECC's version was cheaper than the name brand, too. NECC claimed that they did not just follow, but exceeded, USP General Chapter <797>, the nation's standards for sterile preparations in pharmaceutical compounding. This was reassuring to the clinic's staff. NECC's quarterly "Quality Assurance" report cards showed official-looking results of the company's environmental monitoring and sterility tests. Under "Sterility Testing Success Rate," NECC always scored 100 percent. (Cadden had told the sales force that the quality reports did not "say a heck of a lot," but they said enough.) Culclasure told Schamberg to put in an order right away.

Within months, NECC became the St. Thomas clinic's sole steroid supplier.

E very drug shortage helped the compounding industry grow, but NECC's sales reps were finding that the prescriptions issue remained a sore spot with hospital pharmacists and the doctors to whom they answered. Doctors could not possibly write individual scripts for the thousands of doses they needed to store on-site for future patients and emergencies. This administrative conundrum was a deal breaker for many hospital and surgery center pharmacists.

In one instance among many, NECC had been pursuing a hospital, Winchester Medical Center in Virginia, for years with only a dribble of orders to show for it. When the hospital needed a supplier who could handle the volume of medications they required, in particular an antibiotic solution called polymyxin-bacitracin, NECC finally gained traction. The hospital's pharmacy had been compounding the medication, used to clean open wounds during surgery, itself. But demand grew beyond its own pharmacy's capabilities, even with a staff of fifty. If they could find a traditional manufacturer, they didn't need individual prescriptions for each order. But those suppliers took at least a week. NECC could deliver the drugs in three days. An NECC sales rep met with Winchester's own pharmacy staff to assure them that they could order as much polymyxin as needed from NECC's state-of-the-art lab. (The hospital's pharmacists were even invited to Massachusetts for a tour. They never made it to Framingham, but the offer was reassuring.)

To land a client like Winchester Medical Center, NECC had come up with a work-around for the prescription issue. They would "backfill" the large orders—pharmacy industry jargon for using the names of past patients for future prescriptions. "Unfortunately, we are a 'pharmacy,'" Cadden had once emailed Ronzio, who had asked about backfilling. "How can you get medication from a pharmacy without a prescription, which must contain a patient name? We must connect the patients to the dosage forms at some point in the process to prove that we are not a manufacturer. They can follow up each month with a roster of actual patients and we can backfill. If we just sell drugs, we are a manufacturer." Winchester's pharmacists could write new prescriptions using the names of patients from old records who had received the same drug in the past, or hold off on prescriptions altogether and provide names later. The previous patients' names were listed on the faxed-in order, the hospital got the drugs, and NECC had names to show state regulators, if they bothered to check. At the time Winchester backfilled its orders from NECC in 2011, Cadden had not been visited by an inspector in five years.

Soon Winchester was ordering multiple drugs from NECC, including liter and half-liter bags of polymyxin, sometimes twice a week. The NECC sales department emailed Winchester a long list of products NECC could offer at a cost lower than their competitors. "Hospital Custom Medications. Pain Management. Radiology/ Nuclear Medicine. Surgery. Ophthalmology. Emergency. Over 6,000 'unique' formulations." NECC could do it all. When Winchester's orders grew larger, even backfilling wasn't sufficient; soon NECC just skipped asking for the patient names altogether.

The Sutter Health group in California, a vast organization that currently employs 5,500 doctors at twenty-four hospitals and thirty-six surgical centers, also started placing orders without providing names. Sutter explicitly told Giamei that at the volume they were ordering, it would be too much work for their staff to do so for each shipment. Cadden approved Sutter's request to file orders without patient names.

It was simple math. If the customer ordered enough medications, Cadden would waive the requirement for a patient name, not to mention the other information required of a legitimate prescription—a patient's date of birth, allergies, and other medications they were taking. Some sales reps took another approach. They filled in fake names. Orders for Donald Trump, Silver Surfer, Fred Flintstone, John Grisham, Edgar Allan Poe, Bruce Springsteen, and Tom Brady rolled off the fax machine. Regulators weren't checking, so why not have some fun?

Cadden's strategy to distinguish NECC from his 7,500 competitors was working. Its client roster ballooned: Brigham and Women's Hospital in Boston; Harvard University's teaching hospital Massachusetts Eye and Ear; Alaska Spine Center in Anchorage; Scripps Memorial Hospital in La Jolla, California; Vanderbilt University Medical Center in Nashville; Yale New Haven Hospital in Connecticut. Hospitals needed drugs, fast. Cadden was there for them.

It wasn't always seamless, though. In 2011, the University of Michigan contacted Giamei to challenge NECC's claim that they were regularly testing for drug quality, as advertised. A staffer at the university noticed that NECC had filled an order without providing adequate test results, as required by the USP guidelines. When the staffer asked for them and the sales rep came up blank, the staffer accused NECC of fibbing about being compliant. Giamei worried that Cadden would be annoyed by the contention, but Michigan was a big client, so he emailed the boss:

Hi Barry. On the potency testing, Jamie at University of Michigan is going to potency test this order herself. She had questioned why we do not test as she claims USP requires testing on anything over 25 units, and that our website says we are USP compliant. Don't mean to give you a headache on this, and the conversation went well, but I feel I should give you a heads up on the discussion. Please advise.

Cadden knew the buyer was technically right. While NECC did test *some* of its drugs before shipping them, it did so only in quantities considered insufficient by USP to catch contamination. He emailed back:

We should write that we are 99.999 percent compliant . . . sorry! At some point we just say NO to these nibblers. . . . Unfortunately it was a big $$ order so we let them push us around a little bit more.

Some state pharmacy boards also took notice. That same year, Colorado issued a cease and desist order when it found that NECC was selling drugs without prescriptions in the Denver area. The state inspector alerted the FDA and the Massachusetts pharmacy board—another of at least a half-dozen warnings about NECC made to regulators since 2002. "I would appreciate any information that the Massachusetts Board could provide concerning if this practice is allowed under Massachusetts pharmacy law," the Colorado inspector wrote. Neither agency bothered to investigate.

The backfilling also scared off some hospital pharmacists. In 2012, on a Listserv for pharmacy buyers, one posted: "NECC does not require actual names of patients, we just make up names i.e. Jane Doe, Jack Smith, etc." Michael Blumenfeld, director of pharmacy services at Bellevue Hospital Center in New York, responded to this thread with a warning. "This practice clearly shows NECC is violating FDA guidelines and depending on the State of origin, it might demonstrate that you are in violation of state Statutes and/ or Regulations."

Ronzio forwarded the Listserv exchange to Cadden, who tapped out a quick response on his cell phone. "This guy is a douche . . . + clueless," Cadden wrote. "FDA has nothing to do with compounding regulations. This was all solved and explained years ago. Based on his comments he is really clueless."

Business was booming at NECC, but too many complaints could mean unwanted scrutiny. The sales reps were getting sloppy, saying too much in emails about backfilling and other tricks NECC used, like making up patient names for prescriptions. Cadden leaned on Ronzio to tighten things up. Ronzio had a bellicose style, and when he felt heat from Cadden, he would fire out missives with the caps lock on. In August 2012, he emailed the staff with the subject line: "HUUUUUUUUUUUUUUGE IMPORTANCE," with thirty-two exclamation points.

I know I don't have to say this but also never put anything in
writing. . . . Key words never to say are backfill . . . Or anything along
those lines!!!!

For any reps who did not get it:

Its will be a fatal error for you!!!!!!! (*sic*)

NECC now had dozens of employees, but they were still scrambling to keep up with the orders. Staffers began getting daily requests to work overtime, and weekend shifts were added to the
schedule. The sales reps' regions were changed to take advantage of
time zone differences. Giamei got New Jersey and California, then
Tennessee, which meant he could work a longer day. If he was vis-
iting clients on the West Coast, he'd be up early to talk with East
Coast customers before his California appointments were even
awake. After he was done with the East Coast, he'd still have hours
of calls ahead.

The NECC fax machines that Cadden called his "ATMs" were
in constant whir and clank.

CHAPTER 3

A SLOW-MOVING
MASS-CASUALTY EVENT

DAY 7, SEPTEMBER 24, 2012:
1 CASE CONFIRMED, 5 SUSPECTED

ST. THOMAS OUTPATIENT NEUROSURGICAL
CENTER, NASHVILLE

Dr. John Culclasure felt like crying each time he thought about his gravely ill patients. At least one, Rybinski, was near death. Since Culclasure had received a call from the Tennessee Department of Health one week earlier, five more patients had reported similar symptoms. Four were afflicted with meningitis of an unknown origin, and another had experienced a stroke like Rybinski. Still, Culclasure was confident it was not the injections. In the tens of thousands of epidurals he had done, the few infections he had seen were abscesses—isolated pockets of pus, cured by a fairly straightforward treatment of drugs or surgery. He had never seen a case of fungal meningitis with a corresponding stroke. No textbook, journal, or medical school lecture had ever mentioned anything like this.

Patients who received steroid injections, the kind in which Culclasure specialized, were chronic pain sufferers, many of whom came to his clinic three or more times a year. He developed a friendly familiarity with many of them. His daily routine in the operating room was like an assembly line engineered to keep the patients flowing, along with their insurance payments.

When Culclasure walked into the procedure room, a patient would be facedown on the table, the technician having already prepared the injection site with an iodine solution. Culclasure would pick up a needle and turn on the fluoroscope, a live X-ray machine, to find the exact spot on the patient's back marked by a surgeon. Culclasure told his patients the shot would feel like a bee sting. Then he would inject lidocaine just beneath the skin, then push deeper into other spots.

Once the area was numb, he would insert an epidural needle, always watching the monitor carefully. It displayed the spectral image of his needle inside the patient, moving through tougher tissue near the spine. He would look at the patient's back and then adjust the needle again, his eyes moving back and forth between the screen and the patient until the needle reached the spinal canal. When the needle lost resistance, that meant the doctor had reached the epidural space, filled with fat and blood vessels. A dye called Omnipaque 300 would light up on the screen, allowing him to verify if his needle was placed correctly. If he was on target, he pushed the plunger, releasing the steroid. The procedure usually took six to eight minutes.

When he learned of Rybinski's condition, he'd sought clues that might help explain it. An epidural injection included multiple drugs and pieces of equipment that all needed to be ruled out as the source of the problem. A few days earlier, Culclasure had told clinic staff to call their drug and medical equipment vendors and to check in with patients. A nurse dialed their contact at NECC, Mario

Giamei. She told Giamei that patients at their clinic had become seriously ill. Were other NECC customers reporting similar problems? Giamei replied that he had not heard from anyone else. Culclasure, standing over the nurse's shoulder listening, interrupted. Had NECC tested its drugs for mold or other fungi? Giamei didn't know, but he was confident the culprit was not his product.

Giamei was unnerved. He emailed NECC's operations director, Sharon Carter, to retrieve test results for the batches of methylprednisolone acetate that had been shipped to St. Thomas over the past months. The email would trigger concern from upper management, Giamei knew, so he played it down. "I am frustrated that they automatically assume it is us. . . . I'll bet my last layer of fat it wasn't." Carter emailed back the results they had on file quickly: negative for fungus or any other microbial growth. He forwarded them to the center immediately.

St. Thomas was a good, regular client, and Giamei wanted to do more. He told Ronzio about the incident and booked a flight to Nashville for the following Monday.

Giamei arrived at the St. Thomas clinic the morning of September 24. The lights were off and the waiting room was empty—they'd closed while the state reviewed the situation. Giamei's regular contact, head nurse Schamberg, met him at the front door. They walked through the reception area to her small windowless office. Patients were sick, she said, and the Tennessee Department of Health and the CDC were investigating. "You received the testing data I emailed over?" Giamei asked. She had. Culclasure had scoured it for any mention of a fungal test and found nothing.

Someone knocked on the door—a patient with an appointment. Schamberg escorted the confused patient out, telling him, "We're closed due to an equipment malfunction." The state had instructed St. Thomas to be vague about the sudden closure until they knew more.

When Schamberg returned, Culclasure was with her. He dropped wearily into the seat beside Giamei and started asking questions. Had NECC shipped to other clients the same batches of methylpred that St. Thomas had received? Giamei said that they shipped to more than three thousand customers, and he was sure others had received steroids from the same lots. No issues had been reported. Culclasure speculated that it had to be the needles or one of the other products.

The doctor was particularly worried about a unique needle he used for his steroid injections, which was different from those employed by other doctors at St. Thomas—a butterfly needle with "wings" that popped out to help the doctor steady it. Perhaps the wings had contained mold spores, he said, visibly shaken. If that was the case, he was sure there would be more victims.

"Do you test for *Aspergillus*?" he asked Giamei. *Aspergillus fumigatus* was the species of fungus that had been identified in Rybinski's spinal fluid. Giamei had no idea.

The United States Pharmacopeia standards require that at least twenty vials of a big batch (five hundred vials or more) of a compounded drug be tested—a statistically relevant sample that would indicate the safety of the entire lot. NECC did not comply with this standard; Cadden thought it a waste of product. Instead, the company routinely sent only two vials for testing, no matter how large the batch. It was far from a representative sample, but still allowed him to tout the testing in NECC's marketing materials.

Giamei stressed that NECC's "state-of-the-art" facility held itself to rigorous standards. There is no way it was their drugs. He invited Culclasure and his staff to visit them in Framingham and see for themselves. The doctor did not need to travel to Massachusetts; he believed Giamei. He had been using NECC's methylpred for months with no problems. Like most doctors, he assumed that the drugs he injected into his patients had been verified as safe by *some* standardized body. He would turn his focus to the butterfly needles.

Giamei left the clinic worried and began drafting an email to Cadden and Ronzio while the details were still fresh in his mind. "I continued to reiterate that I was confident our product was not the issue, that he had testing from us to verify that information which was not available from any other source and that we have no other issues in the entire country on this or any other medication." He couldn't stop thinking about how upset and fearful Culclasure seemed for his patients.

Cadden was irate. He called Giamei. "It's going to become a legal matter, and they're going to try and blame us," Cadden said. "We really can't contact the client anymore." Cadden issued a warning email to the entire sales staff: calls from clients about any NECC medicine should be directed to him.

When Ronzio went to Cadden's office to discuss the debacle, the boss looked worried. "It's us," Cadden said. "It's all over. This is my worst nightmare." Ronzio was taken aback: he still did not want to believe that the source could be NECC's drugs. "Well, Barry, let's look at all the other potential scenarios during the procedure. With all the different commercial drugs, the syringes, how could it be us with all the quality systems we have in place, and the test results?" Cadden was silent.

DAY 8, SEPTEMBER 25, 2012:
1 CONFIRMED CASE, 8 SUSPECTED

VIRGINIA DIVISION OF CONSOLIDATED LABORATORY SERVICES, RICHMOND

As NECC and public health investigators scrambled to respond to what was happening in Tennessee, a package arrived in Beverly Jones's mycology lab inside Richmond's public health laboratory building. She slipped on her safety glasses and removed the biological sample.

For nearly two decades Jones had served as Virginia's "one-man mycology lab," as her bosses called her jokingly. She was the guru of fungi. When people got sick from a fungus or mold, the samples ended up here. The background noise in her laboratory was the low hum of a refrigerator housing a rainbow of vials: potato dextrose and other agars, culture media that could coax a fungus into growing big enough to study.

After fifteen years working in a diagnostic bacteriology lab, in 1994 Jones had been assigned to mycology—the one area she hadn't studied in grad school at Virginia State University. She did not take the news of her assignment well. She'd cried. Mycology was quiet compared to more high-profile bacterial and viral pathogens, like the flu, West Nile, and MRSA.

But Jones eventually came around. She'd been chosen for the mycology laboratory because she worked hard and her bosses thought she'd relish the challenge. Fungal diseases were puzzles, and Jones developed a passion for solving them. She worked alone in her tiny lab most days, which was tough at first, but then became a perk of the job.

That day, the sample Jones received came from the cerebrospinal fluid of a forty-seven-year-old man named Doug Wingate. He was a patient in Roanoke who'd been stricken with debilitating strokes after falling ill with a indefinable form of meningitis—although Jones did not know these details. She had been given only the sample ID number and the task of determining its species. All she knew was that another lab had tried, unsuccessfully, to culture it already.

After two days, Jones saw nothing helpful in her petri dish. She tried different foods to promote growth: potato dextrose agar, brain-heart infusion, Sabouraud dextrose agar. She also tried something she had learned in one of her early mycology classes. Sometimes, as she put it, immersing the fungus in nutrient-deficient water, starving it, made the fungus "angry" as it fought for survival. Jones chuckled whenever she described this technique to colleagues. She set about making the fungus angry.

DAY 8: CENTERS FOR DISEASE CONTROL AND PREVENTION, ATLANTA

Dr. Ben Park huddled before a speakerphone in his office, eyes droopy behind his glasses after hours of conference calls. Across from him, Dr. Rachel Smith, who had joined CDC's Epidemic Intelligence Service a little more than a year earlier, jotted notes. Occasionally he glanced out the bank of windows looking over the agency's grassy campus. It was midday and they had already been on a seemingly never-ending rotation of conference calls, the mundane yet crucial busywork of any epidemiological investigator.

They dialed into a call where Cadden and Greg Conigliaro waited. Kainer, the Tennessee epidemiologist, was on the call, along with four members of the Massachusetts pharmacy board that oversaw NECC and the state's public health agency. Cadden's voice crackled greetings over the speaker. The mood was serious but amicable.

So far the investigation had been like walking through a darkened room looking for a tiny object. Since Rybinski's illness came to light, Tennessee's suspected meningitis case count was rising steadily, plus a few more St. Thomas pain clinic patients complaining of headaches and nausea. To rule out possible causes, the investigators had to trace the supply chain for every single item used in each procedure: syringes, anesthetics, surgical dye, the trays that held the medical instruments and vials.

As the first patient, the index case, Rybinski had provided an early clue—the fungus *Aspergillus fumigatus* that bloomed in a vial with the sample of his spinal fluid. Spinal fluid from subsequent patients, however, was not matching his profile; initial tests showed no

Aspergillus. It had been a week since Rybinski's diagnosis, but none of the other suspected cases had tested positive for a fungus. But if it was not *Aspergillus*-caused meningitis, what was it?

Kainer and Park were seasoned disease investigators, forged by their post-doctoral years training in the CDC's elite Epidemic Intelligence Service. Smith was just more than halfway through her two-year stint. EIS officers are like epidemiological Navy SEALs, a nimble force designed to respond when a disease is unusual, or affects a unusual number of people in a community. This means the CDC needs expertise across the sciences, so EIS officers come from a variety of backgrounds: physicians, veterinarians, dentists, PhD epidemiologists, and even environmental engineers.

The CDC and its epidemic corps were born amid global crisis. At the height of World War II, the American South was being devastated by malaria, which is transmitted by mosquitoes. In 1942, the government created the Office of Malaria Control in War Areas, which grew as malaria threatened the health of the general population as well. Once the war was over, the office became the Communicable Disease Center, or CDC. Later, it would be renamed the Centers for Disease Control and Prevention.

This early version of the CDC struggled to define its place in America's peacetime public health system. Another agency, the National Institutes of Health, was already investigating disease outbreaks, but the NIH cherry-picked only the most challenging medical puzzles, and states had few resources to probe the smaller cases. The CDC became their go-to agency.

In the forties, the CDC employed many doctors and scientists who understood vector-borne illnesses like malaria, but few epidemiologists. Epidemiology was still a young field. Johns Hopkins

University had started the first epidemiology department in the world only two decades earlier, in 1919. Most graduates from the program turned down federal jobs in favor of more lucrative and prestigious positions at universities.

A new era at the CDC began in 1949, when a Harvard, Cornell, and Johns Hopkins grad named Alexander Duncan Langmuir became the chief epidemiology officer. Langmuir resolved to create a training program for talented physicians and scientists who might be interested in the field, but had not received epidemiological training in college or medical school. The timing was auspicious, as the Korean War began in June 1950. The U.S. draft provided an exemption for physicians who volunteered to do two years of service in public health. As the war raged on, Langmuir's mailbox filled with letters of interest.

Then an odd disease broke out on the battlefield. More than 3,000 soldiers fell sick and nearly 200 died from what initially appeared to be a flu-like illness that turned deadly. Soldiers became red-faced, vomited blood, and experienced organ failure. There was no recorded history of such a disease in Korea, but Japanese war records described something similar that had befallen Japanese troops occupying northeastern China during World War II. The true cause was never determined, but it was likely caused by the hantavirus, passed on to the soldiers via rat feces in their food. Langmuir, who thought it might have been biological warfare, made his case to the CDC's leadership. What if biological agents were used against U.S. citizens? The country was not prepared.

In 1951, Langmuir enrolled the first class of the Epidemic Intelligence Service, or EIS. Over the next few decades the EIS would have a hand in battling pandemics such as smallpox, as well as more frequent food-borne outbreaks like salmonella and *E. coli*. Its investigators would also help in the fight against uncommon diseases at home and abroad such as SARS, hantavirus, and Ebola.

As the number of cases of meningitis from an unknown cause increased in Tennessee, Park, Smith, and Kainer were among the most prepared doctors in the world to stop it. But not even their elite training could guarantee success. Park still smarted when he remembered how a year earlier, in 2011, he had been investigating an outbreak of mold infections after a tornado in Joplin, Missouri, that killed 161 people and injured more than 1,100. He knew that the pathogen thrived in water, and had advised his team to focus on a reservoir as the source of the fungus, which had been identified as *Apophysomyces trapeziformis*. But they turned up nothing: area soils, not the reservoir, would prove to be the source instead. His mistake, his confirmation bias, had cost the investigation time. He wouldn't let it happen again.

O n the call with NECC, Park asked the questions. Were there contamination issues at their Framingham facility that might explain the meningitis and stroke cases? None, Cadden said. NECC was a compounding pharmacy that distributed its drugs throughout the United States. Its pharmacists usually produced between 3,000 to 5,000 vials of steroids for each lot. They compounded from raw ingredients; NECC was not just repackaging FDA-approved products. And their pharmacists used a large pressure cooker, an autoclave, to sterilize them. This machine should rid the steroids of any microbes, Cadden explained. The pharmacy technicians removed a sample from each lot to send to a third-party laboratory for safety testing, then poured individual portions into small vials. They also had an environmental monitoring staffer who tested regularly for mold and bacteria.

Despite Cadden's reassurances, Smith thought the whole enterprise sounded dangerous. Compounding pharmacies were supposed to make small quantities of drugs based on an individual patient's prescription. This sounded like large-scale manufacturing, with a multi-step process that would provide many opportunities to introduce microbes to the product. In Park's ten years on the job, he had seen other outbreaks associated with compounding errors. His mother was a pharmacist. As a child he had watched her prepare medicines by mixing grape flavoring into cough syrup to make it more palatable to children or adjusting the strength of a medicine for a patient she knew by name. Before he had started at the CDC, this is what pharmacy compounding meant to him. What NECC was doing was something entirely different.

Just months earlier, in fact, Park and Smith had worked another outbreak tied to a compounder in Florida, Franck's Compounding Lab, which made an optical medication that was injected directly into patients' eyes. After a batch became contaminated with a fungus, at least thirty-three people were blinded or visually impaired. The owners of Franck's had refused to talk with the CDC. This time, at least Cadden's confidence and willingness to engage was reassuring. Cadden sounded concerned that the CDC was involved, but he was unwavering: he ran a quality operation. Park thought that both Cadden and NECC co-owner Greg Conigliaro sounded competent and in control. Not only that, they had to recognize that containing any contamination quickly was good for the bottom line. NECC seemed to be aboveboard.

Maybe Park and Smith had a red herring on their hands? Tom Rybinski's case was decisive, but there had been no *Aspergillus* in the other samples. Earlier in the day Park sent an email to his team:

It might not even be a fungus anyway. Maybe we should get the DHQP [CDC's Division of Healthcare Quality Promotion, which investigated infections in hospitals and clinics] to take the lead on this investigation.

Before hanging up, they asked Cadden to send over a list of customers who had received drugs from the same lots, or batches, as the St. Thomas pain clinic. The following afternoon, the email appeared in Park's and Kainer's inboxes. Park double-clicked to open the attachment; in Nashville, Kainer did the same. They scrolled: some 17,675 vials from three lots had been distributed to twenty-three different states.

Park held back a rising tide of panic. There were no confirmed cases outside of Tennessee. But if even a handful of the other vials were contaminated, this was a public health threat of a magnitude and complexity he had never seen.

DAY 9, SEPTEMBER 26, 2012: HIGH POINT, NORTH CAROLINA

Effie Elwina Shaw lay in an emergency room. This was the third time in a month that she had come to the hospital with an unusual migraine. Once again, after hours of waiting, the neurologist on duty recommended Tylenol and prepared to send her home. But this time, her daughter Dawn, a nurse at a country hospital cancer ward, was not having it. Dawn recognized the symptoms of meningitis, a disease that afflicted the cancer patients she saw on a regular basis. It had also killed her aunt Jamie Rie, one of her mother's seven sisters.

The daughter of sharecroppers, Elwina had suffered from back pain since 2007, after her home had burned to ashes. She and her husband, Rex, had lived decades in that farmhouse, and it was full of the memorabilia of a well-lived life. The Shaws had been stationed all around the world with Rex's Air Force postings, and Elwina collected rare and interesting pieces of furniture. Before the fire she had been offered $40,000 for a sixteenth-century desk from a monastery in Spain. It was destroyed in the fire, along with everything else.

Elwina and Rex rebuilt, doing a lot of the work themselves. Even though she was in her seventies, Elwina took on the landscaping, bending over her plants and hauling heavy bricks around the yard so it would look just right. Over time, she developed pain from an ulcerated disk. Medicare required that Elwina go through three steroid injections, a method both cheaper and less invasive than surgery, which is notoriously ineffective. Rex was due for a kidney transplant, and Elwina wanted to get her back fixed as soon as possible so she could take care of him after his surgery. After her final, third injection the headaches started.

In the ER, Dawn, who had worked at the hospital and knew people on staff, insisted that the attending anesthesiologist perform a spinal tap. "We're not leaving here with her," she said. The doctor on rotation knew Elwina from the rural pain clinic where she had received her injections—High Point is a small town. The doctor asked Dawn if she understood what she was asking for; a spinal tap is a painful procedure. Dawn reminded him that she worked with cancer patients. She'd seen spinal taps and much worse. Do it, she said.

The staff turned Elwina onto her side. The doctor pierced her back with the needle, slowly. When the spinal fluid began to drip out, Dawn recoiled: it was milky white. Healthy cerebrospinal fluid is clear. Dawn didn't need to wait for the lab results to recognize the signs of meningitis.

The next morning, a voice mail was waiting for the staff of the High Point Surgery Center, the rural clinic where Elwina had received her steroid injections. It was Dr. Rachel Smith from the CDC. She asked them to call her immediately if they saw any possible meningitis cases and stroke in patients who had received injections of steroids from the New England Compounding Center.

DAY 10, SEPTEMBER 27, 2012: CENTERS FOR DISEASE
CONTROL AND PREVENTION, ATLANTA

Forty-eight hours had elapsed since their call with Cadden. Smith sat at her desk in a beige cubicle in a room with fifty of her colleagues. While the other scientists worked quietly alongside her, Smith had a telephone headset tangled in her hair and was dialing numbers as fast as she could. She had the unenviable but critical task of cold-calling 76 clinics and hospitals around the U.S. that had received those 17,675 vials. She started with those that had received the largest shipments.

The previous evening, the CDC had sent out its first nationwide alert over the Epidemic Information Exchange, or Epi-X:

> On 9/18/2012, the Tennessee Department of Health was notified of a patient with culture-confirmed *Aspergillus fumigatus* meningitis following epidural steroid injection at a TN ambulatory surgical center. Patients have generally received antibacterial antibiotics without improvement. All patients received injections of preservative-free methylprednisolone, preservative-free normal saline, lidocaine, and skin prep with povidone-iodine. . . . To understand the scope of this cluster and identify possible etiologies (sources), we are seeking information on patients with clinical meningitis or possible neurological infection following epidural injections since July 1.

As patients were notified about the alert in Tennessee, those who had received steroid injections began demanding to be tested. A sudden spike in spinal taps created a crush for lab technicians to perform the cultures, and it became clear that the state would need help. That only about 12 percent of the samples extracted from people so far had yielded enough clean fluid to be tested was complicating matters. Each painful spinal tap produced less than a quarter of a teaspoon of fluid, and the amount and quality depended on who was doing the procedure. Emergency room doctors who rarely performed spinal taps were suddenly on the hook to do an increasing number of them, and quickly. This had an effect on testing. An experienced neurologist could get a clean spinal tap with one skin prick, but less experienced doctors often rooted around trying to find the right spot, filling the sample with blood and not enough spinal fluid. Most of the samples coming into the labs in Nashville were not usable.

Dr. Kainer at the Tennessee Department of Health asked the CDC for help, and they quickly agreed. Doctors began shipping vials of spinal fluid to Atlanta overnight packed in dry ice. If the case count continued to grow, as seemed likely, the CDC's labs would be invaluable.

For a new epidemiologist like Smith, the project was terrifying, but also electrifying. She fidgeted while listening to a conference call with Kainer on the latest from Nashville. Kainer's update was important, so Smith ignored the click of an incoming call. Moments later, the click again. So far most clinic directors she'd contacted had been more annoyed at the CDC for asking them to contact patients than they were alarmed at the prospect of an outbreak.

An email marked urgent appeared in her inbox. A doctor from North Carolina had called the emergency hotline with a case matching the description in the Epi-X alert: Elwina Shaw.

Smith hung up and dialed the High Point clinic in North Carolina. A group of clinic staff repeated the information from the email. They were concerned the case was related to those hundreds of miles west in Tennessee. As she listened to the nurse, she sent an email to Park: "Potential case in North Carolina. Getting info now." She was trying to reach the doctor who treated the patient, but he was with someone at the moment, she added. Park shot back: "If you have to, page them."

When the clinic staff hung up, Smith ran to Park's office. She arrived flush-faced and out of breath. "North Carolina," she panted. "*It's so bad.*"

The next morning, the two spoke with Elwina's hospital and epidemiologists at North Carolina's Department of Health and Human Services. Her anesthesiologist told them about Elwina's cloudy spinal fluid and explained symptoms consistent with fungal meningitis. Then he said that she'd had a stroke overnight. Park and Rachel perked up. Elwina's stroke was characteristically similar to Rybinski's. The anesthesiologist happened to also be a partner at the clinic where Elwina had received her injections and confirmed that she'd been given methylpred. The doctor did not think Elwina had long to live. And it wasn't just the steroids that were suspect. The clinic had used the same iodine solution as an antiseptic and the same anesthetic as the Tennessee cases.

The CDC had requested brain tissue and cerebrospinal samples for any new cases so they could see if it was a fungus matching the one in Rybinski's body. Rybinksi would be moved into hospice care and die within days. If Elwina's family consented to an autopsy, samples from her body could be flown to Atlanta quickly.

The request for an autopsy reached Elwina Shaw before she died. Her other daughter, Anna Allred, worked as a hospital chaplain, and had been against the idea. She saw it as intrusive and disrespectful. Elwina sat up in her hospital bed and told everyone except Anna to leave. "You and I have to talk, and then we have to pray," she said. Anna had participated in many deathbed conversations, but this was her mother. Anna had an aversion to autopsies after a particularly difficult visit to a morgue during her chaplain training.

"You have to accept that this needs to be done," Elwina told her gently. If her body could provide clues that might save other lives, they should not stand in the way. Anna delivered Elwina's wishes to her family. They signed the papers.

E lwina's samples, along with Rybinksi's and a few others, were delivered to the lab of an esteemed CDC pathologist, Dr. Sherif Zaki. Unlike Jones's small lab in Virginia, Zaki's lab was state-of-the-art, its hallways decorated with framed photographs of some of the pernicious microbes he had battled over the years. In 1992, Zaki was involved in the discovery of the hantavirus, which caused severe pulmonary infections and initially had a mortality rate of 50 to 60 percent. After 9/11, he had also worked on the anthrax attacks.

The samples of brain and spinal tissue arrived fixed in a solution called formalin and embedded in a wax block. Scientists cut slices off the block to examine under a microscope. They added blue and red stains that identify bacteria, as well as something called Grocott's methenamine silver, or GMS, stain, which identifies fungi. Rybinski's sample immediately turned a deep red. He had had an aneurysm, a kind of ballooning, in the arteries of his brain. Zaki noted a fungus and recognized it as *Aspergillus*.

Zaki moved on to Elwina. The blood vessels of her brain tissue were also inflamed. Something was different than Rybinski's sample. In fact, the fungus from her sample did not look similar at all—it was elongated, with sectioned-off chambers and scars on the ends where its reproductive spores detached. Describing the microbe's unusual branch-like structure, Zaki noted in his report that there were "rare fungal" structures. He could not identify it by sight. The CDC would sequence its DNA along with samples collected from other patients and try to find a match.

DAY 10: RICHMOND

There it was. The water agar Beverly Jones used days earlier had indeed made the mold angry.

She held her dish up for a better look. The half inch of mold that had grown was not blue-green like *Aspergillus*. Mycologists use terms like *woolly, suede-like, cotton-like,* or *glabrous* (smooth or leathery). This fungus was soft like suede. The sample was placed onto a slide using two long knitting-needle-like tools from beneath her worktable. She inserted the tips into a tube with a torch flame to sterilize the ends, slipped on white sleeves and gloves over her lab coat, and placed the petri dish into a ventilated sterile workbench called a hood. She used her needles to tear the mold into smaller pieces and stuck a chunk on a slide. She added blue dye, then squashed the sample below a second slide. At her microscope, she took a closer look.

At first Jones saw only a bird's nest of black hairlike strands. This told her nothing. She turned the slide over. *Boom.* There was something ghostly and glowing in the blue dye. She zoomed in. It looked like a translucent pea pod or a see-through worm. Inside the wormlike body were separate chambers, and at the end of it were scars, where the fungus's reproductive spores had detached as it multiplied in her dish.

She'd seen this fungus before, in samples from patients in Virginia with sinus infections. While the CDC pursued DNA identification, Jones and her colleagues had recognized it almost immediately. Jones had more details about the mold in an old mycology book she kept on a shelf in her small lab. This fungus ate grass and corn voraciously. It was not a well-known human pathogen. There was no literature showing that it had ever caused meningitis, let alone strokes.

The CDC had just sent out its Epi-X alert, and Virginia's health officials suspected the samples she was studying had come from a patient—Doug Wingate—with a profile similar to the ones in Tennessee. In public health, it didn't get any bigger than a CDC investigation. They also said that one patient had tested positive for a common mold, *Aspergillus fumigatus*. Jones called in her supervisor, asking her to look through the microscope and confirm Jones's finding. "This ain't no *Aspergillus*," the supervisor said with a chuckle. Jones nodded in agreement.

CHAPTER 4

BULLETPROOF

BOSTON

Inside a concrete hospital tower on the banks of the Charles River, a woman screamed. She was in the middle of optical surgery, but the anesthetic injected into her eye socket had failed to numb the pain. It was not supposed to happen this way at Massachusetts Eye and Ear hospital, a teaching facility for Harvard Medical School. In March 2012, for the second time that year, the eye block—an anesthetic administered to block a cluster of nerves and numb an area of the body—was not working. The surgeons and anesthesiologists who administered it called their pharmacy manager: what the hell was going on?

Mass. Eye, as it was known, had once made its own anesthetic. But two years earlier a salesperson from NECC convinced the hospital's pharmacy that the compounder's products would last longer than those made in-house. While the hospital's normal eye block expired after twenty-four hours, NECC claimed its product could sit in a fridge for a month because the company tested the drug for sterility. This was a major time-saver, and safer. Instead of having to mix three separate drugs in-house for each patient, NECC's drug was pre-mixed and tested, the doctors thought. That meant that the hospital could see up to sixty ophthalmic cases a day, five days a week. Plus, even though NECC was a pharmacy, Mass. Eye's staff did not have to provide prescriptions or patient names. On their order form, under *Patient's Name* they could just write "per agreement," the NECC saleswoman explained, plus the name of the head of their anesthesiology team. They could do this even though the doctor listed had never signed it and did not oversee the bi-weekly orders for hundreds of prefilled syringes.

Mass. Eye reported the ineffective drugs to Cadden's operations chief, Sharon Carter. Carter asked if Mass. Eye was refrigerating the drug properly. They were, but sometimes staff took the syringes out early to bring them to room temperature, which was more comfortable for the patient. Those few minutes at room temperature should not have mattered; the active numbing agent, lidocaine, did not need to be kept cold. Nonetheless, Carter blamed user error by the hospital staff, and Mass. Eye placed another order.

When they called back a couple of days later with another complaint about ineffective eye block, Carter was defensive. She had checked the worksheet. She emailed:

> The weights of each ingredient are accurate . . . The technician that made your eye block has been compounding for many years and also makes other facilities' eye block as well . . . I understand that you will be ordering 300 more syringes and would like to receive them as soon as possible. I will be looking for your new order.

Still, with multiple complaints NECC agreed to further test the lots to see if there was a problem. NECC sent five syringes for potency testing. A few weeks later, Carter emailed again. The eye block had indeed tested subpotent for lidocaine, containing only 23 percent of what it should have had. Carter noted matter-of-factly that the problem "was due to human error" and promised to start testing each lot before shipping it out, which NECC should have been doing all along. Dr. Sunil Eappen, whose signature had, unbeknownst to him, been on each order, responded to his pharmacist: "What is NECC? It does seem like something that we need to report to the FDA? Does the manufacturer know? What will they do?"

But Mass. Eye's pharmacist, Jo Stewart, didn't want to report the incident to state regulators or the FDA. She felt protective of her fellow pharmacists. Hospital leadership told her to report NECC to the Massachusetts Board of Registration in Pharmacy anyway. NECC had put their patients at risk. She agreed, but first contacted Carter to give her a collegial heads-up. Cadden called Stewart and apologized. He promised that NECC would do a thorough investigation.

A few days later, the state board sent a letter to Cadden. They asked for a list of prescriptions and patient names for the eye drug orders. Cadden called Stewart again and asked for a favor. She didn't have patient names for each drug used, either, but she could send him an operating room schedule with names of everyone who'd undergone eye procedures, and they could backfill the names. Cadden and Greg Conigliaro set out to create a log of prescriptions, adding doctor names where needed.

For the first time in five years, the Massachusetts Board of Registration in Pharmacy had a reason to inspect NECC. Given the board's low staffing numbers, they chose instead to perform a faster "desk audit." An inspector would review the records Cadden and Greg Conigliaro provided, but would not actually visit.

Even so, Cadden was livid. He called his chief pharmacist, Glenn Chin, into his office. From now on, Cadden said, all drugs would be held in quarantine at least seven days. No drugs could ship out until they received clean test results for each lot. "Bulletproof." This is what NECC needed to be. He repeated it so Chin would get the message. *Bulletproof.*

THE NEXT DAY

NECC, FRAMINGHAM, MASSACHUSETTS

Owen Finnegan pulled into the parking lot, guiding his black SUV past the piles of mattresses and old furniture sitting just outside the sterile room where he worked each day. At 7:00 A.M., it was already in the mid-seventies, the sky bright blue, the breeze light. He was in a good mood. He'd just returned from his honeymoon in Bermuda and was feeling refreshed and ready to get back to ten-hour days filling vials of methylpred and other drugs.

Finnegan's vacation bubble popped as soon as he entered the lab and spotted his boss, Glenn Chin, asking for everyone's attention. Chin was tall and often profane—Finnegan joked he was prone to bouts of "'roid rage." Now his face was flushed and he looked angry. "We are changing our testing policies. We need to be bulletproof," he said. "When we send samples for testing, we are not to ship any drug to customers until seven or fourteen days out. We need to appear to be on the up-and-up with regulators."

Finnegan's fellow technician Joe Connolly spoke up. "We've been in business for years, and we're just now coming up with a testing policy?" There was an awkward silence as they waited for Chin to respond, but he just turned and left. After the meeting, Connolly pulled Chin aside. "You know, this testing policy is only going to last until Carter has to call a customer and tell them that an order is going to be delayed."

The next day, Connolly received a recipe sheet for lidocaine that had *NEW FORMULA* scrawled on the page. A clinic in Hawaii had ordered a new formulation and needed a hundred vials. The order was to be made and shipped to Hawaii that very same day. Chin had said that all drugs were being held for potency and contamination testing for a week or two. Connolly called Carter and asked her to double-check the ship date with Cadden.

From his sterile workstation in the clean room, Connolly could see through a window into Cadden's office. He watched as Chin and Carter entered. After a few minutes of discussion, Chin came over. *Process it and send it out.*

Cadden's "bulletproof" drug testing policy had lasted less than a day.

B y the summer of 2012, the orders poured out of NECC's fax machines faster than ever. The company had only about forty-five employees, so Cadden did not yet have the staff to make, fill, package, label, and ship all of the orders coming in. He was marketing NECC as the largest compounding pharmacy in America. And he was under pressure to keep increasing profits. Each family member-owner had a lifestyle to uphold. The majority owner, his sister-in-law Carla Conigliaro, and her husband and NECC founder Dr. Douglas Conigliaro were buying a $4.2 million penthouse in Boston. Greg Conigliaro and his wife, Cynthia, purchased a $2.35 million vacation home on Cape Cod. Of course, Cadden and his wife, Lisa, had their own growing empire, cars, a boat, and multiple homes to maintain.

NECC's employees needed to feel that same urgency. Cadden emailed Ronzio and Carter:

> **The lab downstairs is the engine of this car and we are the gas. They are working extremely hard to keep up with all our orders and we need to show them the same dedication.**

Cadden worried that employees would not step up. They were paid hourly and did not share in the skyrocketing profits. Convincing them to give up weekends and evenings to fill orders, performing the rote jobs of crimping lids on trays of drug vials and stuffing boxes for shipping, was difficult. "I would like to see who volunteers but if we do not have enough, it will have to be mandatory," he continued. "This is the business that we are in and we need to do whatever we need to do to take care of these clients."

The company's sudden growth had meant that Cadden needed help. Earlier in the year, he'd assembled his co-owners and top managers for a brainstorming session: Ronzio, Doug and Greg Conigliaro, and Sharon Carter. They did a SWOT exercise: strengths, weaknesses, opportunities, and threats. Cadden jotted down "Just beginning to scratch surface" at the top of his notes. Under that he scribbled: "Hospitals. Very little competition at this point. Sales 'just' getting some momentum."

The PowerPoint file titled "Weaknesses" included "disgruntled employees, dependence on low-end workforce, size of facility/lack of defined work areas, lack of end product testing, and Massachusetts regulatory environment (strength?)." Cadden was still not sure about the last point, but had good reason to feel like he had it under control. The family had strong ties with pharmacy overseers—NECC and Ameridose's vice president of regulatory affairs, Sophia Pasedis, who also served on the state's pharmacy oversight board.

Near the top of the list of NECC's weaknesses Cadden noted what would turn out to be a critical one: "Recycling center next to facility."

JUNE 29, 2012: THREE MONTHS BEFORE PATIENT ZERO

When Finnegan got to work, Chin was already there. They were preparing to mix one of their moneymakers, a batch of methylpred, and Chin was the man who made it. They checked bins filled with vials of their most popular drugs, which Chin liked to keep in stock so if an order came in they wouldn't get "caught with their pants down." If anything was low, Finnegan would start his day restocking.

They moved into an anteroom and gowned up. Windows overlooked the clean room, a roughly 4,000-square-foot aseptic space where a dozen or so employees made sterile drugs. Finnegan stepped on a sticky mat to remove any debris from his shoes, stretched a "bouffant" over his short hair, put on a mask, and wiggled into a bunny suit. Then he reached into a no-touch washing machine, which sprayed cleaning solution around his hands and forearms. The process took about eight minutes.

Parts of the room's shiny, pale green floors were patched with

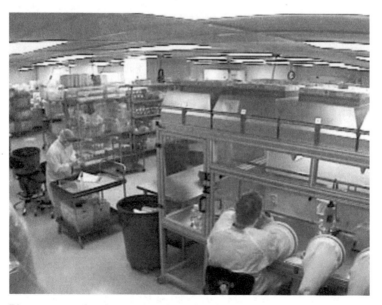

Pharmacists and technicians work in the clean room at the New England Compounding Center facility in Framingham, Massachusetts, in 2012. *(Courtesy of the U.S. Department of Justice)*

trash bags or cellophane secured by duct tape. Sometimes oily goo of an unknown origin oozed through cracks. NECC had been built atop an old train repair depot, where years earlier there had been a significant oil spill. It had been classified by the town as a hazardous waste concern, which could be why Greg Conigliaro got a good price on the property—with a promise to remediate the spill as part of his purchase agreement. As far as Finnegan could tell, though, the trash bag triage was the extent of any action taken. To fix it would interrupt production. (Once, Cadden wrote to the property manager to complain that the oil needed to be wiped up every hour or two. "We will need to jackhammer this area and block this fissure with some sort of cement," Cadden wrote. The property manager had a better idea: "Can we sterilize it and put it into oral dose syringes? I'm sure Ronzio could find a market for it!")

Finnegan stepped over the trash bags and cellophane and powered up his computer to check for orders and play some music, his eyes irritated from the alcohol fumes and latex. The room was a cacophonous mix of music and the drone of air whooshing through filtration. The batch of methylpred on the docket meant there would be thousands of vials for him to fill and prepare.

He sprayed the vials and stoppers he'd be using for the methylpred that day with alcohol. At least once a month he used a product, Spor-Klenz, to combat mold and other fungal growths on his workspace, gloves, and the pump, too. He stuck his arms into the sleeves of his flow hood—a sterile workbench that used filtered air to protect against contamination—to begin work.

Early mornings in the lab, Finnegan often saw something moving in his peripheral vision. Most of the time it was an insect on the floor or crawling on a table or shelf—a long, hairy centipede was the most common intruder. He or another tech would spray it with alcohol until it died. There were also ants, spiders, and mice. Finnegan and Chin knew that insects in a clean room indicated a contamination threat, but the presence of these creatures was so common that after a while they forgot about it.

After high school, Finnegan had played junior hockey for the Boston Junior Blackhawks. He was not a great skater, but he was burly and always willing to fight. He fit in well at NECC since joining the company two years earlier. Chin had hired him after a short interview process. Finnegan had been the lead tech at a CVS pharmacy for a couple of years when he spotted the job listing. In their interview, Chin seemed more interested in how Finnegan would adapt to the company culture than in how skilled he was at handling medicines. "It seemed more like a personality quiz," Finnegan told his father after. "Well, you definitely have one of those," his dad responded. He would also earn more money than ever before, since NECC had raised him to $22 an hour, plus overtime. The most he could make at CVS was $18.

On his first day on the job, Finnegan met Cadden. "I hope you have a thick skin," Cadden joked. Finnegan loved the testosterone-fueled ribbing; it reminded him of the camaraderie of his time playing hockey. With a few other techs, Finnegan started a recreational hockey team, the NECC Soaring Pigeons. Finnegan went to Connolly's house every week to play Dungeons & Dragons, drink beer, and complain about work. Connolly was the best man at Finnegan's wedding.

But the locker room atmosphere sometimes boiled over. The radio was a particular lightning rod. The technicians wrangled over whether they should listen to sports or music in the sterile room. One day things got more heated than usual. Steve Lutz, whom Finnegan considered one of the best pharmacy techs, wanted to listen to indie music. Chin kept tuning into 98.5, the Sports Hub. There was a vote, and the majority went for sports radio. Lutz quit on the spot.

At the time Finnegan held a low-level position, blending eye drops and other lower-risk medications. When Lutz left, a crucial job was suddenly vacant: filling vials and syringes with methylpred and other injectables—those medications they compounded that had the highest risk of causing harm because they are injected directly into the sterile spaces of the human body. Vials came in larger orders, so took more time, focus, and experience. After Lutz stormed out, Chin looked to Finnegan to step up. He said that another pharmacist would help train Finnegan and get him up to speed.

But when Finnegan showed up the next morning, he was on his own. Under USP safety rules, Finnegan should have been put through a series of tests, called media fills, to determine whether his aseptic technique was rigorous enough to take on such detailed work. Pharmacist Gene Svirskiy was busy filling orders of cardioplegia, the heart-stopping drug used in cardiac surgeries. Finnegan had never filled large batches of high-risk sterile drugs before. Maybe he'd done a handful of vials to help out, but not thousands at a time. He asked for help, but Chin was too busy producing the drugs. He didn't have the time to teach Finnegan. Filling methylpred became Finnegan's job.

Just like that, what Finnegan called his "wicked pissah" hours— the consistent eight-hour days, Monday through Friday—were gone. Weekend stints were common. Once he was gowned up and in place, workdays were stressful. Every minute counted. And he was anxious about the risks involved with his new gig. Even a swipe of a sweaty brow or an itch meant you were supposed to don new gloves or wash up. Chin made sure to remind him regularly: If something goes wrong, it could really "fuck someone up."

The chattering of the sports radio helped to keep the other workers from cracking. Long hours each day of wearing goggles, masks, and gowns and being surrounded by the same people led to claustrophobia. So they pranked each other. They wrestled. They sprayed one another with alcohol. They pushed each other through the lab on wheeled carts, making funny noises. One time Finnegan and some others lifted a smaller technician onto the room's conveyor belt, which moved him through a small opening that the pharmacy used to send its drugs out to the shipping staff.

Women did not last long in the clean room. One of the company's only female pharmacy techs, Ashlie Tucker, was forced out after breaking one of Chin's clean-room codes: she complained to Cadden. Tucker, who is black, said she endured racist, sexist banter and offensive jokes. Cadden went to Chin afterward, not to scold, but to warn him. Chin pulled the male employees aside. No more jokes, no more rap music with offensive lyrics, until they could build a paper trail on Tucker to get her fired. That was Cadden's directive, Chin told them. Tucker quit a couple of weeks later, and the chaos resumed.

Skilled, experienced techs like Tucker and Steve Lutz resigned. But NECC was on the rise and needed to hire more technicians, or a "trained monkey," as Cadden once called them, who could fill orders. Some lasted just a few days. A guy from the shipping warehouse came in to help out and stayed. With all the back and forth, keeping the clean room sterile was a steep challenge. Humans are host to trillions of microscopic residents, many of which drop from our bodies as we move through the world. Most are not harmful, but if a microbe makes its way into injected drugs, it can kill. Battling this transfer is a never-ending war. NECC had two clean rooms, with a couple of dozen people coming in and out every day.

Despite washing up and wearing protective suits meant to contain contamination, the fraternal crew that Chin had assembled regularly shed hair and skin. Cadden broached the subject with Chin in an email. "What do you see as the source for the tumbleweeds + hairballs?" Chin responded: "Yeah, there's a lot of hairy zoo animals in the room . . . it's more of the curlier hairs, like the pubics. . . . The cleaners told me this month that the anteroom is actually cleaner than inside the clean room. . . . Joe killed a fly inside the clean room Thursday am."

"U can deal with cleaning procedures + hairy animal grooming!" Cadden wrote back.

But Chin's chief concern was to keep pumping out the drugs. He had been making methylpred for Cadden since 2004, but not under such pressure and time constraints. There were many steps in compounding a batch, each with its own contamination dangers. When Chin arrived each morning, a tech would have gathered and weighed out all the key ingredients for the "base solution" he needed to get started. This included polyethylene glycol, sodium chloride, water, polysorbate 80, and two types of sodium phosphate—everything except the active pharmaceutical ingredient, methylprednisolone acetate. The non-sterile mixture prepared by the tech was run through a sterilizing filter, then left in a foil-covered beaker inside Chin's laboratory glove box.

Chin's chief responsibility was to take non-sterile agents and make them sterile—the most difficult and highest risk of all pharmacy compounding. First, Chin put the beaker with the prepared base solution on a spin-plate inside his glove box to blend the ingredients. As it rotated at high speed and created a vortex, he mixed in a non-sterile methylpred powder along with sterilized water. Next, he pulled the beaker into a small machine inside his glove box, a homogenizer, which used intense pressure to decrease the size of the ingredient particles. Each lot he made held a little more than three gallons, or between five and six thousand doses.

When he finished with the homogenizer, Chin moved the mixture back to the antechamber, covered it with foil again, and removed the beaker from the glove box. He put it into the autoclave, which resembled a microwave oven, where it pressure-cooked for fifteen minutes. The U.S. Pharmacopeia called for a minimum of twenty minutes, and more for big batches, but Cadden and Chin thought that fifteen was sufficient. It saved time. Many pharmacists put a stick called a biological indicator into the oven with the drugs, which contains a bacteria that is known to be hard to kill. When the meds come out, they check to see if the bug died, as evidence of sterility. Chin did not bother to use biological indicators.

After the mixture was autoclaved, Chin moved it back into the glove box and sprayed it down with alcohol again. Using a foot pump, he drained it through tubing into two-liter bottles. He siphoned out the two vials to send to an outside lab for testing: one for the drug's strength, the other for sterility. Again, the two vials were well below the twenty-vial standards listed in the U.S. Pharmacopeia's rulebook.

Chin sent the final mixture to Finnegan to be squirted into individual vials. Sometimes Finnegan ran out of methylpred and could not finish filling an order. In these cases, Chin would mix a fresh batch on the spot. But hospital pharmacists got cranky if they sent drugs with different lot, or batch, numbers. They liked continuity. Instead of giving them two different labels for drugs from two different batches, Chin and his techs "botched lots," the term Finnegan coined for combining the two even though no safety testing had been done on the newer batch. Once the two lots were mixed, they affixed the older, tested lot's label to make it look like one.

In the summer of 2012, they were "botching" lots weekly. Finnegan and his fellow tech Joe Connolly grew concerned. Connolly spoke to Chin and just got another shrug of the shoulders. If the "big boss" said to do it, Chin did it.

Annette Robinson was Cadden's insurance policy against contamination. He hired her without an interview after a chance meeting in a parking lot. Robinson had been fired from Ameridose, one of NECC's sister companies, after she had trouble completing tasks due to pain in her hands caused by repetitive stress. Robinson had once worked for the state, testing racehorse urine for the presence of steroids. She had no experience in environmental monitoring, but Cadden saw a way to fill a gap in his workforce and grabbed it. She'd learn as she went along.

Robinson was a small, nervous woman with a childlike voice. She called Cadden "Care Bear" and liked to tell goofy jokes while she moved around the room collecting her samples. Her primary job was to make sure that the busy clean rooms were under control and that drugs were sent out for quality testing on time. This was not easy. Chin yelled at her to leave if she was annoying him, and none of the men took her seriously. She collected samples by swabbing work surfaces with sterile pads. Her swabs were supposed to go into an incubator so that any contaminants could grow, but, initially, NECC did not have one of those. Instead, before the company bought an incubator for her, Robinson put them in the conference room, underneath some cabinets. She'd taken one course in microbiology in college, and NECC offered no other training. When something grew in one of her dishes, she had a folksy, and inaccurate, way of identifying what it was: bacteria were smooth, fungi fuzzy.

Nonetheless, Robinson took her job seriously. Serving as NECC's quality control person meant she was often the bearer of bad news, like when she found a mold "hit" on a tech's hood. The tech would have to take his sterile workstation apart and clean it. She pressed Chin to make sure that all employees read the safety guidelines she had compiled. (Cadden was too occupied managing his burgeoning customer base to worry about updating their standard operating procedures, or SOPs, which cover cleaning requirements, gowning procedures, recalls, and all other lifesaving public health processes.) "Fuck the SOPs," Chin responded in an email.

But Robinson persisted, even though she was subject to constant belittlement from Chin, Finnegan, and the others. She collected samples from floors and hoods, from the air conditioning registers, from the ducts that brought in air from the rooftop, from the techs' fingertips. She developed a color-coded chart to differentiate her findings. She understood that finding a fungus was worse than a bacterium, and harder to get rid of, so mold hits were red.

Yet her petri dishes regularly sprouted the fuzzy growths. On February 23, 2012, she found mold and bacteria in multiple places: eleven mold colony-forming units, or CFUs, in one spot on the clean-room floor; four mold CFUs and nearly a dozen bacteria around the warehouse and anterooms. She took her reports to Cadden and Chin. Chin agreed to have the areas scoured with antifungal cleansers. A week later, the mold was reduced, but a trace of it was still measured there. On March 29, she found a hair with growth around it near Finnegan's hood; another sample filled one dish three-quarters full with mold. Near Hood 1, where Finnegan filled steroids, her air-testing results were often high for mold or bacteria. On July 5, she found woolly "overgrown mold" on shelves and a bin that Chin used to store the methylpred. She again knocked on Cadden's door, only to be shooed away.

Many molds thrive in warm, damp places. NECC's clean rooms were often warm and damp, despite USP guidelines that sterile rooms have humidity between 30 and 50 percent, and a temperature no higher than 60 to 70 degrees. NECC's air conditioning system and HVAC automatically turned off each night at eight P.M. On August 10, 2012, the day Chin made a big batch of methylpred, the humidity in his clean room spiked during the afternoon to over 70 percent. That night, when the room was empty of people but full of stored drugs ready for shipment, all four of NECC's sensors registered humidity of almost 80 percent. Temperatures in the smaller clean room sometimes reached over 100 degrees, the floor slippery with sweat. Once that summer, Finnegan had to stop working in the room after an AC failure led to temperatures of over 105 degrees.

NECC's official internal "action level" for fungi was three. This meant that if anyone found more than three consecutive samplings with colony-forming units in a given area, work should stop there while the equipment was broken down and disinfected. But Robinson's mold alerts annoyed Cadden. In the summer of 2012, he increased the mold action alert to four and the air action level to nine. With a higher threshold, work would be interrupted less often.

Cadden also sought a scapegoat. He emailed his cleaning company, which came in after hours to regularly mop and wipe down surfaces. "I just watched the surveillance film . . . and it was shocking, to say the least," he wrote. "Your employees have obviously not been trained properly or do not care at all. They are actually contaminating my clean room when they are supposed to be cleaning it." The company's contamination control manager called in his cleaning crew, but they insisted that they had been doing the same thing at NECC for years with no contamination issues. The manager asked Cadden to see the video so he could verify it. Cadden never sent it. When Robinson found the July 2012 bloom on the methylpred shelf, Cadden again said he'd watched surveillance video and thought the problem was coming from their mopheads. But the mopheads were specially designed for work in labs; they were processed in a clean room and vacuum-sealed in that same room. They weren't opened until they were in the customer's facility. The company's manager replied to Cadden: "We service 40-plus accounts and we've never had an issue with our mops being contaminated."

The cleaning company offered Cadden a solution. They would bring in a microbiologist to get to the bottom of NECC's mold problem, and also offered to bomb the clean room with antifungal agents. The manager asked if Cadden would share Robinson's testing data so he could study it for clues. But Cadden neither sent the testing data nor agreed to the antifungal cleaning. He did not allow a microbiologist to investigate. He didn't even provide new disinfectants.

Robinson's chart with red marks reported mold hits almost weekly, even as the company's self-reported Quality Report Cards were being sent out to doctors, hospital pharmacists, and surgery centers throughout the United States telling a different, implausible story: 100 percent clean results. Production carried on.

CHAPTER 5

SHADOW INDUSTRY

OCTOBER 2002

ATLANTA, GEORGIA

The packed conference room at the massive Georgia World Congress Center in Atlanta hummed with the voices of pharmacists waiting for Mickey Letson's speech to start. The occasion was the Medtrade conference, held biannually. Letson's talk was titled "Compounding Opportunities," and he was there to teach the pharmacists how to get rich. His company, Decatur-based Letco Medical, sold the raw chemical ingredients that druggists needed to launch a lucrative business.

When Letson came onstage, he was in a celebratory mood, and for good reason. A few months earlier, the U.S. Supreme Court had handed the compounding industry its resounding victory in the *Thompson v. Western States Medical Center* case, allowing them to directly advertise and market drugs.

"The FDA Modernization Act of 1997 covers everything from a federal standpoint in compounding," Letson said. "If you wanna know it, read [it]. When you finish it, forget everything you just read because it's not valid anymore."

Compounding was the future. There were legitimate reasons to compound drugs, but many pharmacy owners were wary of the cost and liability associated with manufacturing sterile drugs from non-sterile chemicals. Letson ridiculed this conservatism; it was costing them profits. Traditional pharmacies earned a 10 percent profit by simply "counting pills," he said. Modern pharmacy had become nothing more than a distribution network for FDA-approved products made by manufacturers like Johnson & Johnson and Pfizer. By mixing their own drugs, Letson claimed, the pharmacists could earn a "minimum 75 percent gross profit." And it was easy. In advertisements published in *The New York Times* earlier that year, Letson had claimed that "anyone can set up a compounding pharmacy."

"Let me tell you a little story of what happened for those of you who haven't followed this case," Letson said. He began his history lesson.

In the 1990s, compounders had expanded briskly. By the 2000s, the industry's growth was even faster, and messy. The government did not track how many compounding pharmacies had popped up, but the best estimates were thousands, with hundreds in each state. Some were small and made drugs for only a few patients with legal prescriptions. But, as the FDA discovered, others were manufacturing drugs and creating preprinted prescription forms that made it easy for doctors to get ever larger quantities. As more drugs became hard to get in times of shortage, these preprinted forms were too tempting for some physicians to pass up.

The FDA first sounded an alarm in 1992. An increasing number of compounding pharmacies were engaging in large-scale manufacturing, and posing "a very real potential for causing harm to the public health," the agency wrote in a guidance document. Behind the scenes, the FDA's staff heard insider stories of drugs being made in dirty back rooms. One day in 1996, someone sent the FDA a photograph of a cardboard box brimming with doses of compounded drugs being stored next to a filthy toilet. The photo became an emblem for FDA staff members seeking tougher action.

The next year, in 1997, Congress passed the Food and Drug Administration Modernization Act, the law that set the industry on a collision course with the FDA. Part of the Act restricted compounding pharmacies from marketing drugs directly to doctors and consumers. Letson explained: "Pharmacists got together and decided 'Hey, this is totally wrong. We're gonna sue the government because this is a violation of our free speech.'"

In 2002, the Supreme Court agreed, ruling that the Modernization Act's ban on marketing and advertising was unconstitutional. After the ruling, the FDA deferred responsibility for the safety of compounded drugs to the individual states, even though most did not have the inspectors to watch over these pharmacist drugmakers. The Supreme Court victory "immediately began to kick the compounding field in gear," Letson said.

"For those of you that have heard you cannot compound a commercially available product, that is not correct today. Make sure everybody catches up with me on that one," Letson said. Without the interference of a federal agency to slow things down, the industry could make its products and ship them around the country quickly and efficiently. Pharmacies began applying for licenses in as many states as possible, sending drugs to pain clinics and hospitals looking for cheaper and more readily available supplies.

And if the money was not a compelling enough reason to get started, compounding could also provide a brush with celebrity. Suzanne Somers had forged a post–*Three's Company* career working with compounding pharmacists to sell "bioidentical hormones" to ease symptoms of menopause and aging; Oprah Winfrey was also on board, featuring the compounded hormones on her show. Letson told his audience that these hormones, as well as drugs for people with chronic respiratory diseases, were the best type of business—repeat customers. He did not mention that the FDA had issued multiple warnings against taking unapproved drugs. Regardless, compounding pharmacies now had a First Amendment right to market them.

Letson ended on a high note: "They [FDA] have not been very effective at getting the compound pharmacy to stop compounding."

As the industry took off, few people understood it well enough to recognize its risks. One person who did was a pharmacist in suburban Chicago who'd become a student of public health at Johns Hopkins. As Letson lauded compounding's future from the stage, she was preparing to warn Congress and the nation about a looming disaster.

W hen Sarah Sellers faced a particularly intransigent problem, she pictured a knot: a tangle of two sailing ropes, one dark brown and the other tan, braided together like a cinnamon bun. The image graced the cover of a beloved book about a problem-solving process that she had studied religiously in graduate school. Most people will tug at a knot at random, which often makes it tighter. A problem solver studies the knot coolly, creates a plan, then pulls the rope in just the right spot to easily undo the tangle.

Sellers understood more about compounding's dirty secrets than almost anyone inside or outside the industry. In the 1990s, while she was earning her doctorate in pharmacy from the University of Florida, a compounding pharmacist had given a guest lecture urging her class to consider a career in his field, telling them they could thus add another zero to their salaries.

She followed his advice and got a job mixing sterile injectable drugs in Gainesville. One day her boss provided her with an instruction manual and containers of chemicals. She searched the label of the chemicals for an indication that the powder had been verified by the FDA as sterile and safe, and saw nothing. Even worse, the packaging of the filter she had been given to sanitize the drugs explicitly said it was non-sterilizing.

Pharmacists, like doctors, take an oath to do no harm. Sellers had just graduated, the pledge still fresh in her mind. "We can buy the FDA-approved drug, and it would be safer for our patients," Sellers told her boss.

Her supervisor balked. "We could do that, but we're not going to make as much money."

Sellers quit. Over the next two years, she worked for two other compounders, each time encountering the same attitude, shrugging off her concerns about what she considered to be threats to patient safety. The industry considered the active ingredients they used to be safe. If there was a problem with one of their drugs, she was told, the doctor who wrote the prescription would be liable, not the pharmacist.

In 1998, Sellers took her concerns to one of her pharmacy professors at Florida, who connected her with officials at the FDA. Sellers's expertise was invaluable. Congress had a year earlier passed the Food and Drug Administration Modernization Act, and the agency selected Sellers to serve on its advisory committee. She worked with industry and the FDA to improve safety standards.

The FDA dissolved the compounding safety committee after part of the Act was struck down in the nation's highest court. Sellers, however, was undeterred.

A HISTORY OF ERRORS

For millennia, apothecaries made most of the world's medicines. In 1820, the first nationwide attempt to standardize the quality of what was hardly a uniform industry was the publication of the United States Pharmacopeia (USP), a sort of drug recipe book.

Since the mixing of medicines was not centralized or regulated, the U.S. Pharmacopeia created a set of standards, albeit one that was voluntary and haphazardly followed. Stories of deaths due to druggist errors made headlines well into the next century.

In 1857, a story in *The New York Times* told an all too common tale. John, a two-year-old, had been sick in bed at his home in Baltimore. The local druggist, Mr. Ernst Leffer, mixed the medicine prescribed by the doctor: "anise seed water, chloride of potash, lemon oil, and quinine syrup." John subsequently died. When confronted, "the apothecary, confident in the correctness of his compounding, took the bottle of liquid and swallowed a portion, when, within three or four minutes, passing into the presence of his wife, he fell and in a short time expired," the newspaper reported. The pharmacist had erroneously substituted "cyanuret of potash" for "chloride of potash," a relatively harmless compound of chlorine mixed with potassium. He had given the child cyanide.

In 1893, a young drug clerk, Thomas C. Nichols, was convicted of manslaughter charges in a New York City courtroom after a customer, Martin Mundt, had come in complaining of a cold and asking for quinine. "He took a dose, and during the night his brother heard him breathing strangely," the *Times* reported. Mundt died. Nichols, who had been unlicensed and employed at the pharmacy for only two days, had given Mundt morphine by mistake. He was "remanded to the Tombs."

In 1906, the United States took a major step toward safer drugs with passage of the Pure Food and Drug Act, which created standards for food and some medicines. But it protected consumers only from adulterated drugs that were mislabeled. Anything could still be legally marketed in your local drugstore, as long as the variation from the Pharmacopeia's recipe was stated plainly on the label. Deaths from pharmacist errors and adulterated drugs remained a significant public health concern for decades. In 1921,

Congress investigated. One of the resulting inspection reports, of a single Connecticut pharmacy, noted that "of a total of 235 drugs examined, 47 were found to be adulterated, below standard, or otherwise illegal."

Then, in 1937, more than a hundred people, many of them children, died in fifteen states, a tragedy that was traced by FDA field inspectors to a pharmacist named Harold Cole Watkins, chief chemist for S. E. Massengill Company in Bristol, Tennessee. Watkins had developed a raspberry-flavored syrup called Elixir Sulfanilamide, used to treat streptococcal infections. The syrup was easier for children to swallow than the previously available powder and tablets. To make the syrup, Watkins dissolved the tablets in diethylene glycol. Watkins and Massengill shipped two hundred and forty gallons of the red syrup from Virginia to California. Diethylene glycol, a main ingredient in antifreeze, caused kidney failure and a painful, slow death for those unlucky enough to have taken it.

One girl's grieving mother wrote a letter to President Franklin Delano Roosevelt:

> Even the memory of her is mixed with sorrow for we can see her little body tossing to and fro and hear that little voice screaming with pain and it seems as though it would drive me insane. It is my plea that you will take steps to prevent such sales of drugs that will take little lives and leave such suffering behind and such a bleak outlook on the future as I have tonight.

President Roosevelt signed the Federal Food, Drug, and Cosmetic Act in 1938. The Act gave the FDA far-reaching abilities to control the manufacture and distribution of drugs, as well as cosmetics and medical devices, and required that drugs be labeled with adequate directions for safe use. It also mandated pre-market approval of all new medications, such that a manufacturer would have to prove to the FDA that a drug was safe before it could be sold. The Act fostered a modern era of industrialized medicine making. Commercial production of so-called wonder drugs skyrocketed. Production of penicillin alone rose from 400 million in the first five months of 1943 to 650 billion units by summer of 1945.

The days of mixing drugs in the back rooms of corner pharmacies largely faded. Pharmacists instead became Big Pharma's distribution network. With fewer producers, extreme profits for manufacturers also paid for research that produced cures for syphilis and tuberculosis, led to the discovery of corticosteroids, and the development of pills to treat hypertension and diabetes.

Pharmacists, however, could still legally distribute some narcotics without a doctor's prescription. It took until 1951 for Congress to update the Food, Drug, and Cosmetic Act to create a federal prescription-only classification. This further established companies like Eli Lilly as the nation's medicine makers. But, as always, there was an exception. Some patients still had a real need for customized drugs, so Congress allowed pharmacists to compound medicines with a doctor's prescription. Lawmakers reasoned that if pharmacists had to have a prescription to legally compound a drug, there was no way they could mass-produce it.

By 1961, the Bureau of Labor Statistics reported in its *Occupational Outlook Handbook* that "compounding is only a small part of present-day pharmacists' work, since many drugs are now produced by manufacturers in the form used by the patient." By the early 1980s, only 2 percent of all prescriptions filled required compounding.

Yet, the practice was largely kept alive by the Texas-based Professional Compounding Centers of America, or PCCA. In the 1980s, PCCA set up the first one-stop shop for pharmacists who wanted to become drugmakers. The company's chief innovation was to repackage bulk pharmaceutical ingredients, often sourced from China and India, to sell to pharmacists. Pharmacy schools had largely dropped compounding instruction, so PCCA picked up the slack. By the 1990s, it launched a series of seminars aimed at teaching pharmacists how to create sterile drugs, like eye drops and spinal injections. PCCA sent its affiliated pharmacists and other industry experts to talk at schools of pharmacy around the nation, including Dr. Loyd Allen, editor in chief of the *International Journal of Pharmaceutical Compounding*. It was Allen who informed Sellers's class at the University of Florida that compounding could add another zero to their salaries. PCCA also sent speakers to Cadden's pharmacy school, at the University of Rhode Island. It sold a software program called the Compounder with hundreds of recipes and instructions, and it offered the necessary chemicals that were the base ingredients for products ranging from cough syrup to methylpred.

After the Supreme Court ruling in 2002, PCCA launched its most audacious push yet: to get more hospitals to outsource pharmacy services to large-scale compounders like NECC. Many doctors remained skeptical because they did not understand that modern compounding could provide common medications they needed in large quantities. So PCCA began training pharmacists and sales representatives in its "FEAR" system: "False Expectations Appearing Real." At the trainings, the reps role-played scenarios to learn how to get past skeptical doctors and hospital pharmacists. The goal was ultimately to ask the right question, like, "Do you ever wish a medication came in different strength or size, or dye free or preservative free?" The sales training materials explained that "No two doctors are alike. Don't pre-judge them, just plant seeds!"

"Get outside the box!!!" PCCA urged. Potential customers were everywhere. "Veterinarians. Dentists. Sports Medicine. EVERYBODY!!!" PCCA even told the sales reps what to wear on calls: a pharmacy jacket or a lab coat. Have a business card. Use a memo pad and pen to take notes. Look smart.

As PCCA grew, so did its need for political influence. Its related lobbying group, the International Academy of Compounding Pharmacists (or IACP, which today is known as the Alliance for Pharmacy Compounding), quickly boasted some two thousand members, which later doubled, and began contributing hundreds of thousands of dollars to industry-friendly lawmakers.

The FDA was in a bind, paralyzed when it came to oversight of compounding pharmacies. The Supreme Court's ruling had been followed by other lower court decisions that muddied what role the agency could take, if any. So the FDA chose to tread lightly due to hospitals' legitimate need for compounded drugs during shortages. To move against the compounding industry would risk affecting the already imperiled supply chain. Plus, as compounding pharmacies proliferated, the FDA's inspectors were scrambling to understand yet another emergent public health threat: generic drugs manufactured overseas. The agency added to its already burgeoning caseload the work of inspecting facilities making millions of vials of generic drugs in India and China. The FDA was overextended and largely chose to focus elsewhere.

By 2010, at least 10 percent of all U.S. prescriptions were written for compounded drugs, up from 2 percent in the early 1980s. Left to ensure safety was a patchwork of state pharmacy boards. Many doctors had no idea that the medications they had regularly prescribed for years could be made by pharmacists working in a converted train depot next to a recycling plant, as NECC had been doing.

As a handful of people inside the FDA slowly sought a path forward to improve safety at compounding pharmacies, the IACP started a legal defense fund to fight the agency any time it tried to investigate a member facility. Barry Cadden was among its donors.

OCTOBER 23, 2003

U.S. SENATE COMMITTEE ON HEALTH, EDUCATION,
LABOR, AND PENSIONS, WASHINGTON, D.C.
When the FDA's compounding safety committee dissolved, Sellers
was dismayed but not disheartened. She considered law school, but
decided instead to study epidemiology. She was a mother of three
young kids, so she enrolled in a part-time master's program in epidemiology and public policy at Johns Hopkins. She wanted to add
the science of epidemiology to her expertise in pharmacy so she
could attempt to measure the public health effects of compounded
drugs.

For her thesis research, Sellers used her industry knowledge and
FDA connections to begin investigating deaths associated with
compounding errors. The industry was not required to report "adverse events," so she worked her sources and started gathering clues.
She quickly found evidence of a number of tragedies. She reached
out to investigative reporters at major newspapers to share her findings. The first story appeared in 2001, after three people had died
and thirteen others were hospitalized from spinal injections of
bacteria-contaminated steroids made at Doc's Pharmacy in North-
ern California. In all, twenty-two people were sickened. Sellers
explained to a reporter how injectables like those made by Doc's
posed the worst kind of threat. "When a drug is injected directly
into the major highway of our whole nervous system, our body cannot defend itself against any impurities."

In 2002, another compounding-related death raised concerns,
after one man died and five others were infected by a fungus in
injectable drugs made at the Urgent Care compounding pharmacy
in South Carolina. But Sellers could not get Washington's attention
until a *Kansas City Star* investigative series covered a pharmacist

named Robert Courtney. Courtney was caught mixing cancer medicines for more than four thousand patients that contained only a
fraction of the lifesaving drugs prescribed.

After the *Star*'s reporting, Senators Pat Roberts of Kansas and
Kit Bond of Missouri asked the U.S. Government Accountability
Office to gather data on the size and scope of the compounding
industry. The data did not exist. The best the GAO could find were
estimates, all from PCCA and its lobbying arm, the IACP. Meanwhile, the FDA launched a limited study on the compounding
industry. In 2001, it determined that 34 percent of samples of medications it collected from twelve Internet compounding pharmacies
failed a test for sterility or drug strength. (Similar tests on FDA-
approved drugs made by traditional manufacturers typically saw
failure rates below 2 percent.) Sellers's plan to publicize the dangers
of this shadow industry gained traction on Capitol Hill.

Senator Roberts asked Sellers to testify in Congress to address
what he considered to be a public health concern. Sellers spent
months preparing, believing a legislative solution was the best option to improve the safety of the millions of doses of drugs the
compounders were producing. In October 2003, she entered the
airy dark wood-paneled room that houses the Senate's Health, Education, Labor, and Pensions, or HELP, committee. Senators were
proposing an amendment to a Medicare bill that would require
compounders to register with the FDA and to report when their
drugs injured or killed a patient.

Senator Bond called the hearing to order. "We have received reports of non-sterile eye drops causing blindness, spinal injections
contaminated with bacteria and/or fungus, resulting in hospitaliza-
tion and, in some cases, death, and children poisoned as a result of
pharmacy compounding errors," he began. "The Food and Drug
Administration has become aware of over 200 adverse events in-
volving 71 compounded products since about 1990."

Sellers sat alone at one end of a long table. At the other end, also facing the committee members, were three serious-faced men who represented pharmacy regulators and industry. When Senator Bond nodded her way, she spoke slowly and clearly to make sure they heard every word. "It is unsettling that at a time when we are concerned about the quality of drugs accessed outside our borders because they may not meet our federal regulatory standards, that we have a flourishing, unregulated drug industry within our own borders.

"Contemporary compounding exploits current lapses in the law," she continued. "Because pharmacists are not required to detect or report problems associated with drugs they compound, the known cases of deaths, injuries, exposures, and recalls of dangerous products are considered tip of the iceberg by public health experts."

Senator Bond looked toward the other end of the table at Dan Herbert, the president-elect of the American Pharmacists Association. The Association was the largest U.S. trade group representing the interests of both traditional and compounding pharmacists. Its position aligned squarely with the IACP's that "there has been no evidence shown to support federalization of pharmacy oversight."

The senator asked if the Association would support any changes to the current system. "Does anybody think we should not have a mandatory federal system of reporting adverse events? Anyone? Mr. Herbert."

"APhA would support voluntary reporting," Herbert said.

"Voluntary, not mandatory?"

"Voluntary, non-punitive."

Days later, Paul Levesque, the IACP's president, would send a newsletter to the group's two thousand members, warning that "issues which threaten compounding pharmacy, such as an amendment to the Medicare Bill . . . still loom larger than ever. IACP must stand united and clear." The newsletter explained how, a month before the hearing, the Texas-based IACP had paid a visit to the Republican house majority leader, Tom DeLay, in his Houston office to bring him "up to speed" on the bill. IACP explained that it had "already targeted" two Representatives, Billy Tauzin (LA) and Marion Berry (AK), in the House, and Senators Chuck Grassley (IA) and Judd Gregg (NH) in the Senate, "for additional Congressional support."

Meanwhile, the senators supporting the bill couldn't find any compounding pharmacists willing to even entertain it. The lobbyists argued that it would threaten patient access to lifesaving drugs and refused to discuss it further. Weeks later, the amendment died without a vote.

In the three years following the hearing, Sellers finished her public health degree. And she continued working with investigative journalists and Public Citizen, the nonprofit consumer advocacy group founded by Ralph Nader, to expose compounding errors around the country. Every time someone was injured or died from a compounded drug—the eighty patients in six states in 2004 with a bacterial bloodstream infection due to a contaminated saline solution, the three killed in Virginia by contaminated cardioplegia—she was motivated to keep pushing forward. Sellers had the scientific training and background to understand the complexities of the industry, and she felt an ethical duty to make it safer. Since information about patient outcomes was hard to come by and is sometimes hidden in nondisclosure agreements that are a part of legal settlements, Sellers gathered evidence wherever she could find it. She squirreled away newspaper articles, made copies of transcripts of talks by industry boosters like Mickey Letson, combed through court documents, and obtained depositions.

In 2006, the FDA was mounting another push for federal legislation, this time with the backing of the celebrated Democratic senator Ted Kennedy of Massachusetts, working across the aisle with Senators Richard Burr and Roberts. Improving oversight of the burgeoning supply of pharmacist-compounded drugs was part of Kennedy's larger push to reform the U.S. health care system. Other lawmakers began to share their concerns about an imminent public health disaster from companies like NECC, which had started successfully pushing its products into hospitals.

The federal push for oversight laid bare a need for experts on the industry's complexities. "Would you like to come work for FDA on the compounding issue?" the email read. Since the amendment had died, Sellers had started doing drug safety consulting gigs and enjoying her life with her family in Illinois. Her work as a source for journalists had helped shine light on the issue and garnered the attention of senators, but there had been no major regulatory changes. An invitation to work for the FDA's Center for Drug Evaluation and Research, or CDER, was a dream job. She could finally push for meaningful change from inside the agency.

Sellers relocated her family to Maryland and reported for work at the center's modern, mirror-glass building. She had been tapped to join a compounding working group. It was a mixture of FDA staff and members of the U.S. Pharmacopeia, the quasi-governmental group that writes the compounding standards.

But it did not take long for bureaucratic realities to turn her elation into confusion. Within months she was pulled from the compounding working group, with little explanation. Her boss told her that "a special interest group has alleged a perceived conflict of interest." No one ever confirmed that it was the compounding lobbyists who complained, but Sellers knew that she was a familiar and likely unwelcome face for some in the industry. She was told that a decision had been made by someone at the Department of Health and Human Services, FDA's parent agency, and she would be reassigned to another department.

And, as it had done with the earlier Roberts amendment to the 2003 Medicare bill, the IACP mounted a full-scale effort to stifle even a discussion draft of similar legislation. Senator Kennedy abandoned compounding reform as a poison pill that threatened his larger health care bill.

Sellers's personal life began to fall apart, too. Her family was living an expensive life in Potomac, which had become less tenable since she and her husband had separated. A year and a half into what was supposed to be her dream job, a corporate recruiter in the Chicago area emailed her about a job with a major pharmaceutical manufacturer that was looking for experts like her to work on drug safety. And they paid very well.

For more than a decade Sellers warned the public about the looming risk of injectable medicines made at compounding pharmacies. It had taken the deaths of dozens of Americans in the 1930s to spur Congress to reform the nation's drug laws, and she had hoped she could prevent another Elixir Sulfanilimide–like tragedy. But she never found the right spot to tug on the knot. The compounding industry had won.

CHAPTER 6

SIX CONFOUNDING CASES

DAY 14, OCTOBER 1, 2012: 2 DEAD, 11 CASES

ANN ARBOR, MICHIGAN

Lyn Laperriere sat in his bed with a bag of ice propped on his head to dull the headache that had descended without warning. He lived with his wife, Penny, and their two Shichon dogs, on an acre of land in a leafy, quiet neighborhood outside Ann Arbor. Quiet except for Lyn's passion: drag racing. Lyn competitively raced his bright yellow 1969 Camaro around the country, and the couple had converted their garage into a professional workshop. When the two first met, Penny had known nothing about racing. But now when they showed up at their home track, Milan Dragway, or traveled for International Hot Road Association events, she was his crew chief.

Lyn stood five-seven, but at 300-plus pounds, he seemed taller. After nearly thirty-nine years as a skilled machinist at General Motors, he'd been forced to retire when the Willow Run auto plant in Michigan closed. His union pension and Penny's work as a bookkeeper enabled them to enjoy a comfortable lifestyle filled with drag racing and his other passion, bowling.

A few weeks earlier, on September 6, Lyn had seen Dr. Ed

Washabaugh at Michigan Pain Specialists in Brighton to get his regular steroid shot. He endured chronic pain due to spinal stenosis, a genetic disease that he had inherited from his mother. There was a bowling tournament coming up and Lyn wanted to be ready. As usual, he was in and out in little more than an hour.

But then Penny had beaten Lyn in a practice bowl, something that had never happened before. He had been unable to focus on the game. Now he was up in the dead of night, and his head was throbbing. Penny drove to the emergency room at St. Joseph Mercy Hospital, Lyn protesting whenever she hit a bump. The doctors administered morphine, and when that didn't work, Dilaudid. The pain pushed through. Lyn raised his hands around his eyes, shielding them like someone under a spotlight's glare.

The ER doctor ordered a spinal tap. Penny winced as the doctor stuck Lyn multiple times trying to find the right spot. "Are you old enough to do a spinal tap? Are you experienced? I want someone who has done this!" she complained.

There was no immediate sign of bacteria in his spinal fluid culture, but the doctor thought it was still the most probable cause and sent Lyn home with intravenous antibiotics.

A few days later, Lyn still had a crushing headache, and the Dilaudid was no longer able to mask the pain. Penny was driving home from the market when Lyn's number flashed across her cell. "I feel like I'm dying," he said. She dialed 911. She described his excruciating headache. "Help, my husband just called and said he's dying."

When she arrived at home, Lyn was already being loaded into an ambulance, headed back to St. Joe's.

The head of the infectious disease department, Dr. Varsha Moudgal, was perplexed. Lyn was one of six meningitis patients in Michigan that had baffled their doctors. Moudgal loved infectious disease medicine, its investigative bent, but these cases were challenging her training. Tests of cerebrospinal fluid showed spikes of white blood cells called neutrophils, which pointed to a life-threatening infection, most likely caused by bacteria. Yet when the lab tested the fluid for bacteria or the second most likely cause, a virus, the results were negative. Lyn and the other patients were being pumped full of antibiotics. It was possible the drugs were pushing the bacterial numbers low enough to affect the results. But they weren't improving.

A week after Lyn's return to the hospital, Moudgal ordered a fungal test on one of the meningitis patients even though the odds of it turning up anything seemed remote. The hospital sent isolates from the sample to the University of Washington, which had a more sophisticated lab than St. Joe's, but the DNA analysis would take ten days with transit time. In the meantime, she had St. Joe's culture its own sample in potato-flake agar. Within three days, a grayish mold nearly covered the entire dish. The hospital's veteran pathologist determined it was a plant pathogen, although not a species with which he was familiar. Certainly he'd never seen it in a human's central nervous system.

DAY 15, OCTOBER 2, 2012: 2 DEAD, 14 CASES

MICHIGAN PAIN SPECIALISTS, BRIGHTON

A light rain fell on an unremarkable strip mall about forty-five minutes west of Detroit. Inside a pain clinic procedure room, Dr. John Chatas prepared a syringe full of methylpred. His patient that day was his own brother, Michael, who lived with persistent spinal pain in his neck. Dr. Chatas had started Michigan Pain Specialists in the early 2000s with a colleague, Lyn's physician Dr. Washabaugh. In a decade the practice had grown to serve hundreds of patients at multiple locations. Chatas injected the steroid into his brother's neck, pushing the drug into the spinal cord.

It had been a week since the CDC had received Cadden's list of the 17,675 vials distributed in twenty-three states, including Michigan, and a week since Cadden vowed to voluntarily recall the suspect lots of methylpred. The steroid had not yet been conclusively linked to the fungal meningitis cases, so the CDC's Epi-X alert to state health agencies and clinics sent on September 26 did not mention New England Compounding Center by name. The CDC had also sent notices to the professional online communities Clin-MicroNet and the Emerging Infections Network to alert more clinicians about the multistate investigation, and it had organized a call with officials in all twenty-three states affected.

The CDC was trying to be as certain as possible about the quickly unfolding facts before releasing specifics, but word started to spread. Tennessee held its first press conference on October 1, sounding an alarm but also not acknowledging NECC's potential responsibility. "This is a serious disease," Dr. Marion Kainer told reporters that day. "There is not a lot of experience in treating this, but we are getting the best experts together." The CDC's alerts and Kainer's news conference piqued the interest of the media. *The Tennessean* in Nashville and local television and radio were the first on the beat. On October 2, 2012, the same day Dr. Chatas injected his brother, *The New York Times* ran its first story about the Tennessee cases on page A19. CNN reported the story later that day.

None of this information had reached Michigan Pain Specialists. The head nurse, who kept her eye on the clinic's fax machine for recall notices, never saw one from NECC. The day after the news about Tennessee's cases, state public health officials called with a warning: Michigan Pain Specialists was among four clinics in the state with recalled vials of methylpred on its shelves. The warning went to voice mail. It wasn't until the next morning, October 3, that another nurse heard the message and pulled NECC's drugs. The clinic compared the batch number on the vial of methylpred Dr. Chatas had used on his brother with those in the recall. It matched.

CHAPTER 7

A HOUSE OF CARDS

A WEEK EARLIER

NECC, FRAMINGHAM, MASSACHUSETTS

There was little reason to be hopeful, but Barry Cadden wasn't giving up. He couldn't. A CDC investigation threatened everything he'd been building for the past ten years. If NECC's drugs had killed patients, the company would be sued and probably shut down. Maybe it wasn't their fault. Or maybe the problems would be confined to just a few patients in Tennessee. Either way, this was too close a call. If NECC survived, Cadden wouldn't allow such mistakes to threaten them again.

The morning before his call with Ben Park and Marion Kainer, he had emailed Glenn Chin. "I want to tweak our testing + process a little as far as the roids," he wrote. "I think that we can tighten up slightly to cover our behind." He tried to keep a sense of normalcy at the office as whispers about the Tennessee cluster spread among the workers. NECC continued to make and ship drugs, including two methylpred orders from the same August batch that had been sent previously to Dr. John Culclasure's clinic: three hundred vials to a clinic in Abingdon, Maryland, and another hundred to a South Bend, Indiana, facility.

On the call with the CDC, Cadden projected total confidence in his product. He told the investigators that his facility was state-of-the-art. Cadden ended the interview with an assurance: NECC would voluntarily recall the suspected batches of methylpred—two of which he'd shipped out just hours earlier.

Massachusetts pharmacy officials were on the call, too. They told Cadden that their inspectors were going to come in the next morning to have a look. When he hung up, Cadden ordered Chin and his staff to scrub down the clean rooms. They pulled trash bins over the bubbling cracks in the floor.

As Cadden prepared, a nurse at a clinic in Elkhart, Indiana, emailed an NECC sales rep with a problem. Her subject line: "Foreign object in solution after drawing up [steroid]." The clinic was concerned about "gray colored foreign" objects in vials, she wrote, which had been noted by doctors twice that day and once the week before. The color was similar to the drug vial's stopper, so doctors thought it might be related. "I wanted to consult with you and inquire whether there have been any other complaints."

When Cadden received the email, it had been just a few hours since his interview with the CDC. Park had asked if any customers had raised concerns. Cadden had said there were none. Now there was this email from Indiana. Cadden did not yet know that a doctor in North Carolina had alerted the CDC to another likely case there. The evidence was increasingly pointing at his methylpred. Just before midnight, Cadden forwarded the nurse's email to Ronzio with two words: "Oh no."

On September 26 at 2:18 A.M., Cadden started calling some sixty clinics that had received the same methylpred batch as the one in Indiana. Altoona, Pennsylvania. Evansville, Indiana. He left voice messages. Marion, Ohio. Edgewood, Maryland. Nassau, New York. Roanoke, Virginia. "We received a complaint from a client late this past evening of potential foreign particulates in a number of vials they received," he said. "We would like you to quarantine this product at this point. We consider this an emergency, so please, if you get this message, transfer to the individual in charge of medications."

He decided there was no point in scaring anyone about the patients getting sick in Tennessee or the CDC's ongoing probe. He never mentioned it.

DAY 9, SEPTEMBER 26, 2012, 1:00 P.M.

Flanked by his three colleagues, Massachusetts pharmacy inspector Samuel Penta approached NECC's glass front doors. There was a NO SOLICITING sign taped beneath the company's mint-green logo. After a few moments, the building's proprietor and co-owner of the pharmacy, Greg Conigliaro, let the men in. Penta noticed the smell of bleach.

The day before, Massachusetts pharmacy regulators had listened in on Cadden and Conigliaro's call with the CDC. Afterward, the board's director sent Cadden an email tagged "Importance: high." It asked, not ordered, Cadden to confirm that NECC would voluntarily recall the suspicious methylpred. Now the inspectors wanted to look around. Conigliaro and Cadden walked them to an office where the company had quarantined vials of the drugs still in stock, the ones that had not already been shipped to customers. The vials were piled, hundreds of them, in bins on a table. Penta thought that this was an awful lot of steroids for a compounding pharmacy to be making. The amounts were equivalent to those of a drug manufacturer.

Cadden and Conigliaro walked the inspectors back to the warehouse, located behind the sterile labs. The size of the building, as well as the forklift present to move pallets of drugs, was also an unusual sight for a retail pharmacy. NECC had been doing business in Massachusetts for more than a decade, but the inspectors weren't intimately familiar with it, as it was one of more than a thousand pharmacies for which the small team was responsible. None of them were qualified to enter and inspect the clean rooms, which required a special certification and training. Instead, they peered through its windows, where they saw workers in white bunny suits, masks, and goggles, wielding spray bottles and scrubbing away at the tables, shelves, and equipment.

The inspectors returned to the conference room with bins of quarantined steroid vials from the lots that had been sent to Tennessee. Penta held up a bagful for a better look. Since NECC was technically a pharmacy, Cadden would need hundreds of individual prescriptions to be making this quantity of drugs legally. Cadden handed Penta a piece of paper with a list of names and a signature that he claimed was from a doctor. He had never seen a prescription like it, if that is what it was. Cadden also showed the men a pile of documents that indicated where the drugs in the three suspected lots had been sent.

The inspectors spent three hours inside NECC and noted lots of red flags in their official summary, but they did not shut production down. The team was used to going into CVS or Walgreens to ensure that the pharmacists and techs doling out pills were following proper protocols. NECC was something totally different. For the moment, Cadden could continue shipping drugs as long as they were not the products under investigation.

When Penta got back to the office and reviewed the documents, he understood the sheer quantity of recalled steroids that NECC had already shipped. The state board had legal jurisdiction, but it was now clear that the scope of the case was just too massive. The state inspectors were not trained in how drug manufacturers work.

They did not know how to identify adulterated or misbranded products. They were not experts in the laws governing drugs that crossed state lines. They were in over their heads, and they knew it. It was time to ask the FDA for help.

Back at NECC, employees sensed impending doom. Some had seen the inspectors walking around, although no one had given them details. Christopher Leary, a pharmacist who worked with Chin, emailed his fiancée with the subject "big problems." "To make a long story short, there was a huge disaster here yesterday. 10 patients in the hospital with fungal infections from what we think is tainted methylpred," he wrote. "FDA is going to be here in the next couple days . . . which is very very bad."

The next day, in Maryland, Dr. Ritu Bhambhani saw the recall notice that had come over her fax machine. Her pulse quickened. She performed 1,200 steroid injections a year in several Maryland medical clinics, and all the methylpred she used was sourced from NECC. One of her patients had died recently after an injection. The patient had been diagnosed with meningitis and suffered strokes. Within another day or two, Bhambhani had heard from a second patient with meningitis-like symptoms. She had scoured their records and X-rays but could not find anything amiss. When she saw NECC's recall, it did not seem like a coincidence. She called the phone number listed on the fax and spoke to Cadden.

"Oh, it's nothing to be concerned about," Cadden told her. "We're just being overly cautious in recalling the meds." Cadden did not mention what he'd learned from the CDC or the calls he'd gotten from Tennessee and Indiana. "No patient problems reported," Bhambhani jotted on the recall notice.

Just outside of Minneapolis, in the suburb of Maple Grove, Michelle Gieske also received a recall notice. She was the nurse manager at a pain clinic that performed methylpred injections regularly. The clinic had two full-time doctors and one part-timer, and Gieske oversaw a staff of about thirty nurses. It had received two batches of drugs that were being recalled.

But there was something odd about this recall. Usually these notices came with more detailed information—a legal requirement for drug manufacturers under FDA oversight. Since NECC was not federally regulated, Cadden was able to choose the information he wanted to release. It mentioned something about particles found in a syringe, but there was nothing specific about what the clinic was supposed to do with the patients who had already received some of the recalled medication.

When Gieske arrived to work the next morning, she called Cadden. He explained that a concerned nurse in Indiana had alerted them to some "floaties" in a syringe. The nurse, Cadden continued, had reported that she believed the problem was in the plunger of syringes they were using, not in the drugs. He reassured Gieske. "At this point, just monitor your patients," he said. It had been less than forty-eight hours since Cadden had spoken with the CDC about the deaths in Tennessee. "Nothing needs to be done," he said.

Despite Cadden's encouraging words, Gieske decided to do her own detective work. She and her nurses pored through patient records to identify who had received shots from the recalled batches—some eight hundred patients. In the coming days, it would take an entire staff effort working through the weekend to reach them all.

The next day she called Cadden for an update. He never called back.

DAY 9: NECC, FRAMINGHAM, MASSACHUSETTS

Owen Finnegan and Joe Connolly were gowned up and filling vials when Chin interrupted. Stop production and scrub, he said. They cleaned until the end of their shifts. As they left for the day, they saw Annette Robinson with someone they did not know enter the clean room and start collecting samples.

Half of the next day, too, was spent scrubbing hoods, scraping the rust off the steel carts they used to move equipment around, and mopping. After a couple of days, Chin finally let some information slip. It was time to "cover their asses," he said. Some people in Tennessee had gotten sick, and NECC products were a possible cause.

Later Finnegan and Connolly huddled with their colleagues to speculate on what was happening. Anyone could be in trouble. Each considered themselves careful and skilled at their jobs, with good aseptic technique. They started pointing fingers, speculating about who was sloppier. Connolly referred to another tech who everyone thought took shortcuts. "I think I mentioned last week about his mopping, how he turned an hour-and-fifteen-minute process into a twenty-minute process," he continued.

Later Finnegan was taking beakers out of the autoclave when pharmacist Gene Svirskiy came over. "Just so you know, some people are going to be asking about your filling techniques today," Svirskiy said. Finnegan was taken aback. "What the hell does that mean?" Svirskiy was vague. "I just want to give you a heads-up."

Finnegan had filled many of the vials that had been recalled. He walked over to Chin. "What the hell is Gene talking about?" Finnegan asked. "Don't worry. We'll get to it. We'll talk about it later," Chin responded.

Finnegan worked, his stomach in knots, the rest of the day. No one ever arrived to interview him, and Chin never mentioned it again.

DAY 11, SEPTEMBER 28, 2012: STONEHAM, MASSACHUSETTS

Inside the spartan New England district office, FDA investigator Stacey Degarmo read an email from the Massachusetts state team looking into NECC. They wanted help with the investigation. Degarmo's office had inspected NECC at least twice over the past

decade—first in 2002, after the company's steroids had given patients meningitis-like symptoms, and again in 2004 after complaints
from pharmacists. The FDA's reports noted unsafe conditions for
making sterile drugs, and its inspector had notified Massachusetts
regulators. The FDA had issued warning letters. Since then, NECC
had largely disappeared from both agencies' radars.

Now NECC was again in the center of a cluster of illnesses. This
request for FDA assistance was a second attempt since the outbreak
began. Seven days earlier, Dr. Ben Park had been the first person to
send the agency a heads-up, but it hadn't connected. "Vanessa, if
you're not the right person to direct this to, please let me know," he
wrote. Even though the FDA and the CDC reside under the same
federal umbrella, the U.S. Department of Health and Human Services, communication between the two is not streamlined, and
Park's email to his contact had bounced back. As the breadth of the
disaster became clear, the CDC was still trying to get the information to the FDA.

But as FDA inspectors prepared to go in after the Massachusetts
request for help, they were held up. "We are working getting clari-
fication on our inspectional authority," wrote Amber Wardwell, the
New England District's compliance branch director, in an email to
staff. A public health emergency was unfolding, but the FDA was
frozen, unsure whether its inspectors had jurisdiction in Massachusetts.

FDA inspections of traditional manufacturers are wide-ranging
affairs to ensure that drugs are being made under Current Good
Manufacturing Practices. For a compounding pharmacy to meet
CGMP standards would require registering with the FDA, millions of dollars in facilities and equipment, and regular inspections.
This was the red tape the compounding industry had fought so
hard in court and in Congress to escape.

Degarmo's team waited four days while the FDA's lawyers figured out what to do. As they debated, NECC continued to ship and scrub the labs. Finally, FDA and Massachusetts pharmacy officials agreed that an FDA team would look for unsafe conditions that could have led to contamination, and Massachusetts inspectors would accompany them.

Degarmo was pregnant and could not go into NECC's clean rooms, with a possibly deadly pathogen in there. As soon as she got the go-ahead, she texted Almaris Alonso, a Boston-based FDA microbiologist with three years' experience at the agency: "Get ready for an inspection tomorrow." When Alonso arrived at six A.M., she learned that she'd be taking microbial samples of the facility.

DAY 14-15, OCTOBER 1-2, 2012: 2 DEAD, 14 CASES

The first thing the federal inspectors saw as they pulled into the parking lot was a huge mechanical shovel tearing into a pile of decomposing mattresses, construction debris, and trash. Degarmo watched dust kick off the junk as the machine chugged away.

Inside, under the office's fluorescent lights, she acquainted herself with NECC's business operations, to understand the scope of what Cadden was doing. She picked up some of the vials of methylpred that had been pulled and saw what looked like white cotton fibers inside others.

She read the labels. Many simply listed the client name instead of an individual patient. Some read "no patient names required." Did NECC have individual prescriptions for these drugs? she asked. Cadden handed her a folder full of papers, explaining that they used preprinted order forms in compliance with the federal prescription requirement. To help customers save time, Cadden said, hospitals or clinics provided lists of names, and NECC personnel transcribed them onto prescriptions.

Degarmo took a closer look at the documents. She wanted to

know if NECC was making their methylpred with the same ingre-dients as the commercially available versions. Since compounding pharmacies were not FDA-approved, they had to make "custom-ized" versions, from unique recipes. Cadden explained that they made methylpred without a preservative, which differentiated it from the commercial variety. Later, he mentioned that the com-pany shipped 95 percent of its products to other states. *This is not a pharmacy*, she thought. *It's a drug manufacturer.*

D egarmo's colleague Alonso met with Annette Robinson. It was clear right away that Robinson was unqualified to be the quality assurance chief, beginning with her limited education in the field. When Robinson explained how she differentiated a mold from a bacterium—"The fluffy ones are molds"—Alonso had tried hard not to scoff. Not only was this unscientific, it was inaccurate, as bacteria can also appear filamentous.

"How many mold hits do you get a year?" Alonso asked.

"Five." She flipped through a binder with Robinson's environ-mental monitoring reports and noted more than five hits just over the past nine months. Each time, Robinson had sent an email to Chin or Cadden, but there was no indication that NECC did follow-up testing or extra cleaning—both requirements of USP General Chapter <797>, the industry standards Cadden had proudly plas-tered all over the company's brochures.

When Alonso toured the small changing area connected to the clean room, she noticed that the floor mat used by staff to clean debris from the bottom of their shoes was strewn with strands of grass. She didn't have her cell phone with her, so she tapped the arm of the state pharmacy inspector and asked him to take a picture with his.

She crouched for a closer look and saw what appeared to be wheel tracks across the mat, the same size as the wheels of the carts that the pharmacists used to transport boxes of supplies into the clean rooms. If a cart rolled across the mat, picking up the dirt, and grass, its wheels could quickly be covered with fungi and bacteria.

Later in her inspection, Alonso zipped on a gown and affixed a respirator mask tightly over her face. She covered her hair with a hood. Chin and Robinson didn't bother with such precautions, but for all she knew, there might be a killer fungus inside. They accompanied her as she used a sponge to collect her samples, moving methodically around the room and wiping different surfaces. When she finished with each sponge, she dropped it into a sanitized bag that contained a culture media. At one of the autoclaves, the oven that sterilized NECC's drugs, she noted that it was covered in a black-brown muck. She brushed it lightly with her sponge.

By six P.M., the long, focused hours Alonso had spent in a full body suit had taken its toll. Alonso looked at Robinson and said, "I feel chilly." The clean room was at the recommended 60 degrees, and she was wearing only the thin gown over her clothes. Robinson joked, "Don't worry. At eight o'clock it's going to get hot because they shut off the air conditioning."

Alonso snapped to attention. Shut off the air conditioning? This was a shocking revelation and Robinson did not seem to realize it. NECC had agreed to let the FDA in, but with strict time limits. Alonso was supposed to finish her inspection by day's end. Now she needed more time to gather the company's records showing the clean room's humidity and temperature overnight. The company's lawyers were starting to show up, and the FDA was not sure how much longer it would have before the inspectors were asked to leave, as was NECC's prerogative.

The next morning, Alonso hurried to arrive at NECC early and meet with Robinson, who had the air monitoring records. Alonso made copies of as many as she could. Later, when she reviewed them, the overnight data consistently showed spikes in the clean rooms' humidity starting at 8:00 P.M. and ending at 5:00 A.M.—the exact times Robinson said the AC was turned off. The room where NECC made its medicines was a hotbox.

DAY 16, OCTOBER 3, 2012: 2 DEAD, 18 CASES

When the inspection teams arrived for a third day, they couldn't go inside. They were to wait while the state negotiated a temporary surrender of NECC's pharmacy license. This interrupted the FDA's investigation: under the agreement its lawyers struck with the state pharmacy board, the FDA couldn't go in without the local team. The microbial tests and other work would have to wait.

Degarmo and Alonso sat in a car with their colleagues behind a Walgreens, bored and anxious to get back inside. The inspectors had seen foreign objects inside some vials of methylpred that were visible to the naked eye. They would ultimately identify similar visible traces in eight out of one hundred vials that they spot-checked.

Pressure was building. More sick people were being identified every hour. The FDA team needed to get the drugs to a lab for testing. They had vials with visible contamination, but they required lab analysis to confirm it. The FDA's limited jurisdiction meant that they required permission from NECC to remove anything from the premises. If they took the vials without the proper authorization, they could jeopardize their evidence in any future legal action.

They had to get permission from the company right away. In conversations with the FDA's inspectors, Greg Conigliaro had held steadfastly to his conviction that NECC's drugs were not the cause of the outbreak. As a co-owner, he could give the FDA the vials to prove that they were clean. His family, however, had begun to panic. They would have to surrender the pharmacy license during the in-

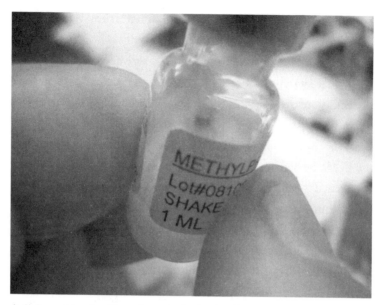

A dark smudge of mold can be seen in a bottle of New England Compounding Center steroids seized by the U.S. FDA in October 2012. *(Courtesy of the U.S. Department of Justice)*

vestigation, and were looking at bankruptcy if their drugs were at fault. Greg's older brother, Doug, and his wife, the majority shareholder Carla, who had nearly $20 million in the bank, began a series of transfers of millions of dollars, and hundreds of thousands in cash withdrawals.

As they waited to reenter NECC, Degarmo's team sent a release request to Greg Conigliaro. She was careful not to mention that they had seen anything suspect. Before the end of the day, he agreed to give them ninety-eight vials. Neither she nor Alonso got back inside that afternoon, but the methylpred came out.

JAMAICA, QUEENS, NEW YORK CITY

Philip Istafanos was on alert for incoming samples from Massachusetts. All the veteran FDA microbiologist knew was that they were tied to a big case. His supervisor drove from New York toward

Framingham while another FDA consumer safety officer drove with the vials from Framingham to meet halfway.

The drugs, all from the August 10 lot, arrived at his lab around seven P.M. Istafanos rolled a vial between his fingertips, scanning the milky methylpred inside. There was something else in there, too, a black particle of some kind. He eyeballed the ninety-eight vials; the same muck was visible in nine. In nearly three decades at the FDA, he had never seen anything like this with the naked eye. It would take weeks for Istafanos to finish testing all of the samples, but within hours of receiving them, he could confirm that they were tainted just using his microscope. He alerted the investigators.

Under the microscope, he saw multiple cells tangled together. Bacteria are prokaryotes, which means their cells don't have a nucleus. Molds are eukaryotic and can be made of cells that have a nucleus. These fungi were bundled into tubes with multiple arms, or filaments.

Istafanos worked steadily into the night. He removed half of each one-milliliter vial and divided the cloudy liquid into two petri dishes, each with a different nutrient broth. He put the last drop from each vial on a plate with an agar of malt extract, where it would grow quickly if fungi were present. Within five days, a black fuzzy mold was spreading from the middle of the malt extract. In the center of the cloud was a pinkish-beige color that indicated a yeast. It would be the same in forty-nine out of fifty petri dishes; all but one sample had both mold and yeast, and one grew yeast only.

As Istafanos raced to confirm the presence of fungi, state officials, confronting a wave of sick and dying people, grew impatient with the guarded federal response. Neither the FDA nor the CDC had yet to publicly name NECC as the likely source. States with an increasing caseload, like North Carolina, wanted answers. On the day Istafanos tested the vials, an official with the North Carolina pharmacy board emailed the FDA.

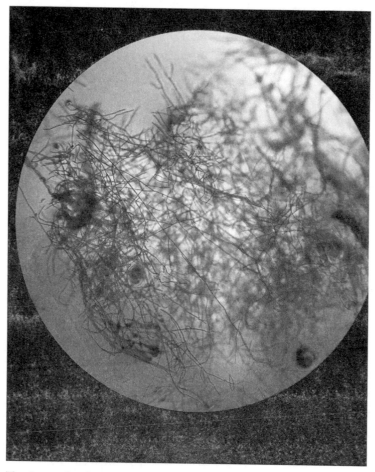

The fungus found in New England Compounding Center's steroids, as seen through the microscope of a U.S. Food and Drug Administration scientist in October 2012. *(Courtesy of the U.S. Department of Justice)*

Patients in North Carolina have been harmed and are at risk. I need to take some action here. So if FDA cannot disclose even the identity of the suspected compounding pharmacy, I'll have to go my own way on this thing. Unfortunately, I'm not in a position to sit around for several days while FDA debates internally about what information to release.

Back in New York, Istafanos's work was just beginning. He also unpacked the forty-one environmental samples collected by Almaris Alonso, added a fungal broth, and set them out to incubate. FDA inspectors had mentioned that NECC cleaned before her samples were taken, so any microbes may have been injured. But bacterial and fungal contamination is tough: many microorganisms are hard to eradicate even with harsh cleansers. They're survivors. In Istafanos's lab, the microbes could repair their cells, grow, and multiply.

After a few days, and despite NECC's cleaning efforts, eleven of the forty-one samples grew bacteria and molds. On a sample from the vent return that sucked air from the clean room, Istafanos found a mold that looked similar to what he had seen in the vials. He scratched out rudimentary drawings of the long hyphae, or threads. On other samples he found multiple species of spore-forming bacteria known to be resistant to disinfectants, along with another mold with banana-shaped spores, a pink yeast, and more.

Dr. Ben Park's team at the CDC received the initial results from Istafanos's laboratory with both shock and relief. It had been about two weeks since the first meningitis case had cropped up in Tennessee. Thousands of Americans, in twenty-three different states, were at risk. It was time to alert the public.

CHAPTER 8

OCTOBER DELUGE

DAY 17, OCTOBER 4, 2012: 5 DEAD, 35 CASES

CENTERS FOR DISEASE CONTROL AND PREVENTION, ATLANTA

Dr. Park spoke slowly into the phone. He now recognized how widely NECC's drugs had been distributed, and he had the FDA's confirmation of contamination. He felt unsettled. This was unlike anything he or the CDC had ever dealt with, and there were still a lot of unknowns. The CDC estimated that 13,534 patients had been exposed. The number of dead and sick was rising by the day. The still-evolving case definition being used to identify at-risk patients included symptoms of meningitis in people who'd also received an injection of NECC's methylpred. Did the mold in the vials match the fungus inside the patients? Also, they had still not confirmed the species of fungus. There was a 40 to 50 percent mortality rate in the patients they knew about. Yet Park thought there was still a small chance they were about to name the wrong culprit.

Listening in were a gaggle of reporters, from *The Tennessean* and *The New York Times* to the Associated Press. Park started with a brief description of what had been happening in Tennessee, and how the testing of patients' spinal fluid had been negative until a fungus was discovered in one sample.

"On September 28, 2012, investigators identified a case outside of Tennessee, possibly indicating contamination of a widely distributed medication. To date, a total of thirty-five cases in six states have been identified with a clinical picture consistent with fungal infection. Tragically, at least five deaths have been reported. Fungus has been identified in the specimens obtained from a total of five patients thus far." Since Park had learned of the case in North Carolina—the first non-Tennessee case—the CDC's outreach efforts found others in Virginia, Florida, Indiana, and Maryland.

He paused. "While investigation into the exact source of these infections is ongoing, all infected patients received preservative-free methylprednisolone acetate from among three lots voluntarily recalled by the New England Compounding Center in Framingham, Massachusetts." It was the first time that the company's name was publicly linked to the investigation.

Symptoms, including the strokes, were manifesting one to four weeks after injection. Park told reporters that he believed what they had seen so far was likely to intensify. NECC had faxed recall notices for the three lots of steroids, but the drugs were distributed so widely that there was no guarantee word would reach doctors and nurses. The drugs had been distributed throughout nearly half of the country. Park read out the names of the states: California, Connecticut, Florida, Georgia, Idaho, Illinois, Indiana, Maryland, Michigan, Minnesota, North Carolina, New Hampshire, New Jersey, Nevada, New York, Ohio, Pennsylvania, Rhode Island, South Carolina, Tennessee, Virginia, Texas, and West Virginia.

What was once a cluster of cases was now an outbreak. The media in the affected twenty-three states started alerting the public. The

CDC opened up its Emergency Operations Center, which is used only during pressing public health threats, most recently a year before, after the earthquake and tsunami in Japan that inundated a nuclear plant and caused a meltdown. The control center's monitors flickered on, with neon-colored maps tracking the state-by-state spread of known cases. Fifty staff members flooded in initially, and would grow to hundreds, all CDC employees reassigned from their normal posts. They made their way down call lists of potential victims. Vats of coffee were wheeled in.

The effort would be the largest direct-patient outreach in the CDC's history, dovetailing with the efforts of state health departments in Michigan, Indiana, Tennessee, Virginia, Florida, New York, and the other affected states, where health care workers, law enforcement officers, and volunteers raced to dial each patient.

ALBANY, KENTUCKY

The call took Joyce Lovelace by surprise. The woman from the outpatient clinic where Judge Lovelace had been treated for back pain the previous summer wanted to know how he was doing. They had a patient with an unusual disease and were doing a routine follow-up. "Well, he passed away," Joyce said, confused. The caller offered condolences before hanging up.

A few days later, Joyce mentioned the call to her daughter, Karen. Her mother's story rang a bell. Karen had seen a report about the alert from the Tennessee state health department and had reached out to her father's doctor to inquire about his shots. As her mother relayed the message from the clinic, the details struck Karen as similar to the state alert—headache, nausea, and strokes in patients who'd received a steroid injection. Her father had been buried with "unknown cause" on his death certificate. This meant that Eddie's family could not collect his life insurance, which did not cover death by old age or illness, just an accidental or untimely demise. None of them believed the healthy judge had died so suddenly without cause, but they seemed to have no recourse.

Joyce decided that her husband's body be exhumed.

NECC, FRAMINGHAM, MASSACHUSETTS

As clinics and hospitals around the country scrambled to sequester any NECC drugs in stock, a dour mood fell over the company. The day before the CDC's big news conference, Owen Finnegan had arrived at work at his usual time of 7:30 A.M. In the break room, he and Joe Connolly had started putting their stuff into their lockers when they saw Chin getting into his gown. His face was bright red, a color it always got when he was upset. Finnegan looked at Connolly. "Uh-oh," Connolly said. Chin saw them watching and drew his hand like a knife across his throat.

"We need to get gowned up," Connolly said. The pair hurried to get into the clean room where Chin was waiting, their colleagues gathered around a table. Chin looked like he'd been crying. "We're doing a voluntary shutdown," he said. "I'm so sorry this is happening. We're going to shut down today. There's a meeting soon. Break the clean room down. We're having a meeting with Barry. I'm sorry. I'm sorry this happened."

Forty-five minutes later, the employees crowded into the break room in front of the wall of lockers. Cadden and Greg Conigliaro entered with a woman from Human Resources. Five patients had been "hurt" at a clinic in Tennessee. The company was going to voluntarily shut down during the investigation, which would likely take two weeks. Employees would receive an email in a week with a restart date. "We'll be back up and running as soon as possible," Cadden said. "I don't want anyone to worry. Your jobs are all set," he added.

Greg Conigliaro spoke next. "Just remember, you all signed a confidentiality agreement."

Many of the employees filed to the bar across the street. Finnegan decided to go home instead. He sensed that things were worse than Cadden and Conigliaro were letting on.

As he was driving, Finnegan's phone rang. It was Chin. "Hey, Glenn, what's going on?" Finnegan said. "You guys are over at the bar?"

"When the media comes over, you can't talk to them," Chin said. Finnegan said he wasn't at the bar. Chin hung up abruptly.

It wasn't until Connolly turned on the television after dinner that night that he learned about the outbreak. He felt his heart in his stomach. Five people weren't hurt. They were dead.

DAY 17: ST. JOSEPH MERCY HOSPITAL, ANN ARBOR

Three days had passed since Lyn and Penny Laperriere's happy retirement was sharply curtailed. They were in Lyn's hospital room in one of St. Joe's dense brick towers when Penny saw the news crawl across the muted television in the corner. It went by quickly, but she noted the words *meningitis outbreak*.

Lyn's doctors were huddling just outside the room. He'd developed bleeding around his brain stem. Penny broke into the conversation and told them what she had just seen. Lyn gave her a skeptical look, and the lead doctor also noted the information without reaction. She took out her phone and looked up "meningitis outbreak." Headlines quickly came up about the CDC's investigation, the possible tie to NECC's steroid injections, and the Tennessee cases. She thrust the phone into a nurse's face. "Look at this!" But the medical team remained focused on Lyn's immediate deterioration and waved her off.

She left the room and found a quiet nook off the hallway. She texted a tip line at Channel 4, which had run the news ticker, and was eventually connected to a reporter. "My husband has all of these symptoms and nobody's listening to me," she said.

Next, she dialed Michigan Pain Specialists, the clinic where Lyn had gotten his steroid shot, and was connected to Dr. Washabaugh. He knew about the recall. The clinic had received a voice message that morning from the Michigan Department of Health and Human Services about it, and the CDC's guidelines for contacting patients. He told Penny that Lyn was injected with a drug that might have been contaminated. "Have his doctors there look for mold," Washabaugh advised her.

D r. Varsha Moudgal learned the answer she'd been seeking for weeks over the car radio. St. Joe's infectious disease chief had tuned in to NPR, as always, during the trip home to eat dinner with her six-year-old son and husband. There it was: the CDC was investigating fungal meningitis cases tied to a possibly contaminated steroid.

At the hospital, Moudgal's colleague, Dr. Anurag Malani, or Anu, was scanning CDC's Health Alert Network email, which had been sent out to health care providers nationwide after Park's briefing.

As of October 4, 2012, five deaths have been reported. . . . These cases are associated with a potentially contaminated medication.
Investigation into the exact source is ongoing; however, interim data show that all infected patients received injection with preservative-free methylprednisolone acetate (80mg/ml) prepared by the New England Compounding Center, located in Framingham, MA.

Both doctors suspected that this could explain their six confounding cases. Most of these patients had been released home after being treated for bacterial meningitis. If they had instead been injected with a deadly fungus, they needed to get back to the hospital fast. The next morning Moudgal and another physician called each one to confirm that they had received a steroid shot in the past few months. One by one, they repeated the same story: they'd been injected at Michigan Pain.

Moudgal notified the Michigan state health department that her team had confirmed the link with the steroids under question. Next, she called Dr. Washabaugh, who was driving the forty minutes to the clinic to join his staff working on notifying patients about the recall. He'd just spoken to Penny Laperriere, and been on his phone nonstop. He'd spoken to the daughter of a patient who had died ten days earlier, checking to see if the death could be related to the news. Washabaugh described the symptoms of fungal meningitis. They matched her mother's case perfectly. She had died with no diagnosis or explanation, her corpse donated to the University of Michigan for scientific research. He told the daughter to request an autopsy as quickly as possible.

Washabaugh's phone rang again. It was an infectious disease fellow at the University of Michigan who had the body of another one of his patients. The fellow asked: Was it possible the steroids that he injected were linked to the outbreak? Washabaugh said yes, it was.

In the course of his drive, Washabaugh had learned that two of his patients were dead. He sat in the parking lot to listen to the voice mails that had come in while he was calling others—all patients who had seen or heard the stories and wanted him to call them back.

Dr. Varsha Moudgal sent Washabaugh patient data related to her meningitis cases that he could use to compare against the list of people he had injected. Now instead of cold-calling hundreds of his patients to check if they were sick, he could cross-reference the hospital network's list to identify those who had developed symptoms. The first familiar name he saw was that of Carol Sakstrup, who had been diagnosed with meningitis in August. He recognized multiple names as his patients. There had been no meningitis cases in the hospital network up until August 2012. Then suddenly all of these Michigan Pain patients started showing up.

Three days after Washabaugh's colleague, Dr. Chatas, had treated his brother's back pain with his regular injection, the state of Michigan sent out a press release saying that six fungal meningitis cases in the state were caused by "potentially contaminated" steroid injections. Michael Chatas endured multiple spinal taps at St. Joe's, which confirmed what he likely already knew: he had a fungal infection.

DAY 19: 7 DEAD, 64 CASES

LANSING, MICHIGAN

Willard "J.R." Mazure was in a good mood. He had just celebrated his fiftieth birthday with friends and family. Mazure had spent most of his days behind a fourteen-foot-tall hammer smashing concrete for a construction company, the shock waves rattling his 230-pound body with each blow. Once he turned forty, the back pain was never totally gone. Because of his job, he could not take opiates, and two surgeries had not fixed the problem, either. Steroid injections worked for about a month at a time. Ultimately he had to give up his full-time union job with its $100,000-a-year salary and retirement benefits. He now took short-term jobs. The shots allowed him to continue to fish, hunt, and even to build a barn on his land.

But with his last shot two weeks before, something felt different. He could swear that there was a *lumpiness* to the injection site, and after the steroids wore off, his pain was ever present.

Mazure sat in the parking lot outside his wife Linda's job at an electronics manufacturer in Lansing, waiting for her shift to end. His truck's radio was tuned to NPR, and that's when he heard it: Michigan Pain Specialists was notifying patients that it had received a batch of steroids that might be related to a meningitis outbreak. It was Friday, and he hadn't heard from anyone at the clinic. On Monday, he got through to a receptionist. She sounded rattled as she riffled through papers. "Your name is on the list," she told him. The clinic had not confirmed whether he received a shot from the contaminated batch, but she would get back to him. She told him a list of symptoms to watch out for: headache, light sensitivity, fever. He hung up. He never got headaches, but now his temples were throbbing. Was it psychosomatic?

The next day, the clinic called back. Since they had talked, Mazure had developed light sensitivity. His neck was also starting to lock up. He didn't like to admit that something was wrong, but Linda got him into the truck and headed to St. Joe's.

When they walked into the emergency room, Mazure saw Dr. Washabaugh. As an anesthesiologist, the doctor had been asked to help out with the crush of patients, many his own, who needed spinal taps. Washabaugh rushed over and touched his face, spreading Mazure's eyes open and feeling around his neck. The look on the usually jovial doctor's face alarmed him. "You got it," the doctor said.

Mazure was given a spinal tap. The pain was intense as the needle went in. His headache worsened. Soon it was official. He had fungal meningitis. The fungus inside him felt different from the back pain he'd gotten used to. Before, his pain was sharp and aching. Now it was a burning, like barbed wire.

* * *

Down the way from Mazure's hospital room, a man with in-tense gray-blue eyes was storming down the hall and out of the hospital.

Ray Gipson had recently retired after nearly four decades making Ford cars at the Michigan Assembly Plant in Wayne. He and his wife of forty-four years, Gayle, lived in a small house off an un-paved road in Ypsilanti, just outside Detroit. Their two grown daughters lived nearby with the grandkids. Gayle had just had a deck built, covered with an awning to protect them from summer thunderstorms. She'd also put a metal swing big enough for two under the tree canopy on their land.

Gayle was devoted to her family and the Church of Jesus Christ of Latter-day Saints. These days she moved her "five-foot-nothin'" frame, as Ray called it, more gingerly due to spinal osteoarthritis. She visited Michigan Pain every three months for a shot of steroids to help squash the chronic pain. Her last had been on August 29. When she emerged, she had been crying. The shots in her spine were always painful, but she never cried. Ray called the clinic the next morning and said the shot was not working.

By early October Gayle's back had worsened. She'd been in and out of the hospital. Ray couldn't sleep. It was the dark early morn-ing, and he decided to check the answering machine. He hated cell phones, so they still had a landline. There was a message from the clinic, asking Gayle to call as soon as possible. Ray had been in such a fog of work and worry from taking care of his wife that he'd not watched television in days. The answering machine also played a friend's voice: they'd seen a report about a problem with drugs at Michigan Pain Specialists. He should check with them immediately.

Ray reached a nurse at Michigan Pain first thing in the morning. He grabbed paper and pen and took notes. Gayle had all the symptoms, from confusion to headache to nausea to light sensitivity. Now she had a high temperature, too. He called an ambulance.

Gayle was put in a small room in the same wing as the other fungal patients. Two nurses tried to get her to lie flat on her bed. As his wife cried out in anguish, Ray yelled at them to stop. They called security. Ray was told to leave the hospital.

DAY 28, OCTOBER 15, 2012: 15 DEAD, 214 CASES

The burgeoning outbreak consumed doctors, nurses, and staff at hospitals in nearly two dozen states. At St. Joe's the hours were long and intense. Dr. Moudgal was missing parent-teacher conferences. Dr. Malani's three-year-old daughter had started asking, "Where's Daddy?"

Malani's meningitis caseload grew from two patients to dozens nearly overnight. The patients came in not knowing for sure if they were infected, and if they were, whether the hospital could cure them. Each death was a blow to the fungal patients who did not know if they'd be next. Each had a worried family with lots of questions. The hospital quickly became ground zero in the national emergency.

And it was just beginning. The construction worker J.R. Mazure, the retired drag racer Lyn Laperriere, the stay-at-home grandmother Gayle Gipson, and the doctor's brother, Michael Chatas, were among 195 fungal patients who were admitted to St. Joe's that October. Each needed a spinal tap and an MRI so doctors could determine if the fungus had colonized their bodies. Some were nearing death; others had no symptoms. Many would never leave. In an information vacuum, the doctors decided to be aggressive, administering two antifungal drugs at once. They were operating without an instruction manual.

The CDC assembled the world's foremost medical mycologists to help guide their treatment, who became known as the "Gang of Six." As the Gang debated heatedly which antifungals to recommend and at what dosage, they grasped one truth: all options had significant, unavoidable risks. Human and fungal cells share similar biological traits, so a poison powerful enough to kill one also damages the other. There were few medicines on the market to combat invasive fungal infections. And they still didn't know exactly which mold they were up against.

One class of drugs, echinocandins, were more useful against yeasts than molds. They were out. The next was the nuclear option, a polyene called amphotericin B. Since its discovery in 1955, it was the only weapon against diseases like fungal meningitis. But it was now given in only the direst cases because of its brutal side effects, including severe kidney damage. It could also be fatal.

Another choice, the azoles, were widely used for human infections like athlete's foot, but also by veterinarians, farmers, and the timber industry. Voriconazole in particular could be absorbed into the human central nervous system, where this mold was thriving. Another plus: it could be administered orally, which meant that if patients needed months of therapy, they could take pills instead of needing an intravenous hookup. It performed well in the lab. But it, too, has terrible side effects, including kidney, liver, and pancreatic damage. Hallucinations were common, as well as nausea, wasting, and hair loss.

As the number of cases grew, the Gang recommended using voriconazole. The CDC instructed doctors to watch patients closely for side effects and to reduce the dosage if severe ones emerged. The St. Joe's doctors had already started with a more aggressive regimen of both amphotericin B and voriconazole, with varying results.

In a matter of two weeks, J.R. Mazure had gone from hunting

and building barns to fighting for his life. He was given 450 milligrams of "amphoterrible" and 450 milligrams of voriconazole each day. The side effects began as soon as the antifungals hit his bloodstream. His body began shaking uncontrollably, which he called "the rigors." He saw ghosts; one night he swore that a dog ran through his room. Another night, he screamed at the nurses that a tornado was ripping through the hospital, tearing off a wall. He was never sure if he was asleep or awake.

A few doors down, Lyn Laperriere, on the same two-drug regimen, had started jabbing at the air. His wife, Penny, asked him what he was doing. "Picking grapes," he said. Soon he broke out in rashes. It turned out that he was allergic to the amphotericin. He stabilized briefly on the voriconazole alone, but was still so weak that he could not raise himself out of a wheelchair.

Around the nation, thousands of people rushed to their doctors to see if they were infected. Hospitals were competing for a dwindling supply of antifungal agents—and no pharmacist would now solicit the help of a compounder. The hospitals instead relied on distributors, the middlemen between them and the Big Pharma manufacturers. St. Joe's also pulled pharmacy and administrative staffers off their usual jobs to call wholesalers in search of the drugs.

With patients coming in almost hourly requesting tests for meningitis, Drs. Moudgal and Malani faced another challenge. How to administer these drugs? Amphotericin B is dripped into the body intravenously, but it is delivered to the pharmacy as a powder that must be mixed a certain way to turn it into liquid. Most powdered drugs take five minutes to dissolve, but this one took fifteen minutes. The doctors developed a step-by-step guide for how to administer the medications, which would change each day or two as they learned more and tweaked dosages and frequency.

Early on, the CDC had instructed doctors to extract 1¼ tablespoons of spinal fluid from each patient—half to count white blood cells, half to culture in the lab—an amount that emerges drop by excruciating drop from the needle. The directive said if the patient's spinal fluid had a white blood cell count of more than ten and there had been an exposure to NECC's steroids, the presumed diagnosis would be fungal meningitis. If the white blood cell count was under ten, the patient was to be sent home and monitored. As the agency learned more about the severity of the disease, it lowered the floor to a white blood cell count of five to ensure that anyone infected was hospitalized.

After the CDC updated the case definition, St. Joe's had to call back the patients who'd been cleared and sent home. Some underwent four or more spinal taps. One day St. Joe's performed more than sixty, and would go on to do more that month than the hospital usually did in an entire year. The hospital called in all the help they could find, including Dr. Washabaugh, his partner Dr. Chatas, and their colleagues at Michigan Pain, all of whom reported for duty alongside the hospital's physicians.

Lyn Laperriere's parents and sister had flown in from Florida. He was tired and flitting in and out of consciousness. The family decided he should rest, so Penny took them out to get dinner and groceries. Lyn leaned against the doorjamb of his hospital room and waved goodbye.

As Penny drove them home from the market, her phone rang. It was the hospital. *You've got to come back.* She felt her face flush, her temperature rise. She ran red lights all the way back to St. Joe's and left the car idling in front, her keys and his family still inside. When she burst into Lyn's room, he was lying naked and bloody on the bed. The doctors had cut his clothes off and were trying to restart his heart, which hadn't beat in nearly an hour. Penny grabbed his arm, screaming, "You can't leave me! You can't leave the dogs!" Nurses escorted her from the room. Lyn's heartbeat came back, but his brain activity did not. Penny calmed down and returned to the room. Lyn's mother was next to Lyn. She put her hand on his face and pushed one of his eyelids open. She looked back at Penny. "He's gone."

R ay fed Gayle breakfast every morning and went home only to shower. He had practically moved in to St. Joe's. Every few days one of their daughters, Rachel or Donna, would come by after they got off of work so that Ray could get a break. It was mid-October and the antifungals were working. Gayle had improved enough to be moved out of the ICU.

Tonight Donna was on duty. Donna had been up for more than twenty-four hours between work and the visit. She wanted to go home to her kids. Gayle asked her to stay. Donna said that Ray would be there in a couple of hours for breakfast. *Just go to sleep.* Gayle begged: *Please stay.* Donna left after Gayle drifted off.

The next morning Ray got the call to come quick. Gayle was being placed on a ventilator. He drove the half hour to St. Joe's, meeting their daughters there. The family had to wait all day to see her as the doctors finished inserting the ventilator. Finally, that evening, the nurse emerged from Gayle's room and told them to go to the cafeteria and get dinner. When they finished eating they were allowed to enter two at a time. They spoke to her, but she couldn't respond with the ventilator in place.

Gayle's doctor asked to see the family in a conference room. She was going to die, although it was not clear, exactly, what from. She had fungal meningitis, as well as kidney failure, perhaps from the antifungals. Now the ventilator was the only thing keeping her alive.

Ray was in a fog. Just weeks earlier he'd been sitting with Gayle on their back porch, and now she was slipping away.

He and the girls went back in. It had been about two months since Gayle's last steroid injection. After the doctors removed the ventilator, she was able to breathe under her own power for a few minutes, but could not talk. Gayle squeezed Ray's hand. He saw only terror in her eyes. Then her hand stopped grasping his, but he wouldn't let go. Donna put a hand on his shoulder. "Dad, let's go. She's gone. Let's go, Dad."

A few days later, Ray and his family sat before Gayle's casket at Uht Funeral Home. The hospital had transferred her body there without an autopsy. If it wasn't required, Ray did not want it. Within fifteen minutes, Ray was summoned by the funeral home director. "You can't bury her yet," he said. "She needs an autopsy." The CDC wanted samples, and now the director told Ray he was

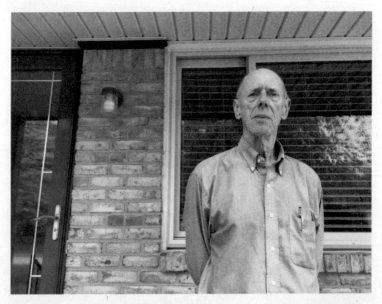

Ray Gipson, whose wife, Gayle, died after contracting fungal meningitis from mold-contaminated steroids, outside his home in Ypsilanti, Michigan, in 2019. *(Courtesy of the author)*

concerned for those of his staff who had embalmed Gayle's body. Had they been exposed to a virulent microbe?

Ray didn't believe his wife's body was contagious. All he'd been told was that Gayle had been injected with a contaminated drug before she died. He was too grief-stricken to put up a fight. The family signed off on the autopsy.

Weeks later, when two FBI agents walked into his backyard, Ray would learn more.

J.R. Mazure lay still in the cavern of an MRI machine, its magnetic imaging equipment chirping, pulsating, and humming. His spinal tap needle had come out covered in fungus. The MRI would give the doctors a better look at a pus-filled abscess at the injection site. In St. Joe's cramped, dark radiology office, doctors sat in front of large computer screens concentrating on the black-and-white images in front of them. They were the first to see what thousands of confounding meningitis cases looked like on the inside.

There on Mazure's scan was a malignant-looking mass sitting in a bundle of his nerves. The fungus had enveloped a vertebra and eaten part of it away. Dozens of patients were also showing these abscesses near the site of their injections. Some did not even have symptoms, but their MRIs revealed the extent of the colonization. Others, like Mazure, had both meningitis symptoms and an abscess. It was a quandary for the doctors. Should they try to remove these fungal masses in patients who did not yet appear to be sick? Or should they wait and see if the powerful antifungal medications worked to eliminate them? Everyone who received an injection would need an MRI. St. Joe's had only two of the machines, so they ordered two mobile ones.

Complicating matters were the intended effects of the steroid injections. Methylpred is an anti-inflammatory that suppresses the body's natural immune response, so many patients had not felt the infection until the steroids wore off over about four weeks. The methylpred itself had provided a cocoon of protection for the fungus to get comfortable in the central nervous system, where the natural immune response to an invader was delayed by the steroids. As he watched the images pop up on his screen, one doctor thought to himself that you would have a hard time concocting a better way to hurt someone.

As was true with the meningitis, deciding upon a treatment for these fungal abscesses would be a conundrum. There was no medical literature on how to handle unidentified fungus living on human spines. The hospital chose an aggressive approach: doses of antifungals and surgery. Specifically, doctors performed decompressing laminectomies, which meant cutting out pieces of bone in the spine to alleviate pressure, and scraping out the fungus using tools that look like tiny shovels.

The normally orderly surgical practice at St. Joe's had turned into a triage center. An incredible 153 people had been diagnosed with an infection at the site of their injection, 112 of them with spinal or paraspinal infections, and the hospital's six neurosurgeons had been working nonstop for a month and a half. When they opened up the first wave of fungal abscess patients, the fungus was pinkish and glistening. One surgeon shouted, "What the fuck is that?" They washed the infected area of each patient with saline solution and then drilled to cut away any bone that was in the way, preventing a clean shot at the fungus. Each procedure took an average of three hours. They worked through the night, each taking up to eight fungal patients. When their colleagues came in the next morning, they'd take whatever cases were left over.

They saw patients whose dura mater, the protective membrane

enveloping the brain and the spine, appeared thick and leathery. In others, it was film-thin, almost see-through. Some of the fungus had made it through the dura into the central nervous system; some of it had not. Perhaps the fungus was hungry to move into the spinal fluid on its way to the brain's blood-rich environment. Equally plausible was that the shot had deposited the fungus both inside and outside the dura, depending on the injecting doctor's technique. It was impossible to know.

Over the next six weeks, St. Joe's surgeons would perform these operations on 116 people. They couldn't be sure the procedures were even useful—this was, after all, uncharted territory—but the hospital administrators believed that they gave patients a better chance of survival, so they recommended them to everyone with a suspected fungal abscess. Michael Chatas, the brother of the Michigan Pain Specialists doctor, had the surgery. J.R. Mazure, meanwhile, would spend seven months in the hospital, undergoing five spinal surgeries. It seemed like they got it all, but there could be no guarantee that the fungus would not return.

DAY 31, OCTOBER 18, 2012: 20 DEAD, 257 CASES

NASHVILLE

Dr. Marion Kainer had barely slept in weeks and was surviving on coffee, adrenaline, and fear. When she did catch a few hours of sleep, it was often on a couch in her office. About a month had passed since she had reported the first case, Tom Rybinski's, to the CDC. It was late on October 18, and her birthday. She stayed up going over mathematical models of patient data that her staff had been collecting since late September. She was close, finally, to answering a question that could help doctors put up a better fight against a disease with an initial 40 to 50 percent mortality rate:

Were patients at a higher risk of infection depending on which of the three batches of NECC's methylprednisolone acetate they received? If doctors had this "attack rate" for each lot that was distributed, they could prioritize treatment for the patients injected with the most dangerous lot.

Since the outbreak's first hours, Kainer had worked toward gathering the raw data she needed to calculate the attack rates. She'd sent her staff to the St. Thomas clinic and others, where they'd faxed each patient's information in to headquarters. They had collected hundreds of profiles this way, painstakingly building their database. But most clinics had not noted which lot a given patient had received, so Kainer's team had to compare the date of the shot with inventory records. About a thousand people in Tennessee had received the contaminated drugs, and the patient database was now substantial enough for a meaningful epidemiological analysis.

The CDC and state health departments were close to notifying 99 percent of the nearly 14,000 people at risk, but they weren't able to provide them with many answers, and antifungal medications were still hard to come by. Now the team finally had the raw numbers they needed. It turned out that, for the Tennessee cases at least, the attack rate was significantly higher in patients from the June lot, followed by August, and then May.

Within days, the CDC released guidelines for clinicians to prioritize antifungal treatments for the people injected with the June and August lots.

DAY 43, OCTOBER 30, 2012: 28 DEAD, 363 CASES

CENTERS FOR DISEASE CONTROL AND PREVENTION, ATLANTA

The index case in Tennessee, Tom Rybinski's, had identified the pathogen as the fungus *Aspergillus fumigatus*, but no subsequent patient had tested positive for it. The CDC's investigators needed to confirm the fungal species before they could finalize their own treatment guidelines, which were still evolving.

Weeks earlier, Beverly Jones in Virginia had identified a mold in the samples that was not known to cause meningitis. Once Dr. Mary Brandt, Dr. Park's boss at the CDC, got the photos, she agreed; this was not *Aspergillus*.

Meanwhile, the CDC's labs were inundated with dry-ice-packed boxes filled with vials of cerebrospinal fluid. The goal was to isolate the fungal DNA and run it through a genetic database to find a match. But first they needed a tool that could reach into a sample and amplify just the bit of genetic material they wanted to study. Working with one, or even just a few, strands of fragile DNA is difficult. But Brandt's lab would make copies of the fungus's genetic code via a polymerase chain reaction, which works like a microscopic photocopy machine, spitting out millions of copies of DNA in about two hours.

A pattern became clear. Sample after sample revealed the genetic bar code of a fungus rarely implicated in human disease. The limited scientific literature that did exist said it was a plant pathogen that ate grasses and corn. There were no known meningitis cases caused by this microbe in previously healthy patients.

Dozens of samples later, they could confirm what many had suspected from the start. They had spent weeks looking for the wrong killer. Rybinski's positive test for *Aspergillus fumigatus* had indeed been a red herring.

The true culprit was *Exserohilum rostratum*.

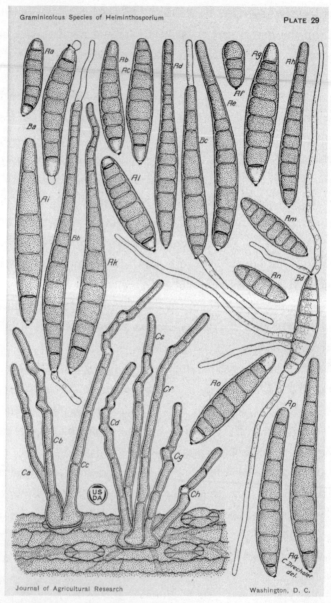

The fungus that would later be named *Exserohilum rostratum* as drawn by Charles Drechsler, the plant pathologist who first described it in 1921. *(Courtesy of the U.S. Department of Agriculture via the Gray Herbarium and Harvard University Herbarium, Harvard University)*

CHAPTER 9

AN OPPORTUNISTIC KILLER

Bloodthirsty—that's how Dr. Ben Park described the fungus. Once injected into some patients' spines, *Exserohilum rostratum* wormed through the cerebrospinal fluid up to the head. In the brain, it ate its way through the blood vessels and grew, choking its host's arteries. Now that it had a name, the CDC scoured the medical literature for any information, but unearthed very little.

The first mention of the microbe that would be named *Exserohilum rostratum* is found in a century-old agricultural journal article written by a Harvard-trained plant pathologist, Charles Drechsler. He noticed the microorganism as a brown splotch afflicting a flowering weed called stink grass. The fungus under Drechsler's microscope had not been previously described. To the naked eye it was unremarkable. But when magnified, it was monstrous, having translucent, almost caterpillar-like conidia, or spores, separated into chambers, with scars at the tips. Its filaments, or hyphae, looked like a clutch of branches that splayed out from the surface of any plant it infected.

In 1921, as Drechsler concentrated his lens on this gangly growth, the scientific world was still coming to terms with what decades later would be recognized as a unique classification of life: the king-

dom Fungi. It is still the least understood of the microbial king-
doms. Of an estimated 1.5 to 5.1 million species of fungi believed
to exist on earth—which include mushrooms, the yeasts that make
wine and beer, rusts, smuts, mildews, and molds—humans have
named or described only about 140,000. Of those, about 300 are
known human pathogens.

In the nineteenth and early twentieth centuries, bacteria and
viruses were discovered to be the source of major diseases like tuberculosis, cholera, and influenza, thus dominating early research.
Fungi were generally categorized as members of the plant king-
dom. Yet scientists like Drechsler knew that parasitic fungi could
sicken other organisms, due to the work of Agostino Bassi, an Ital-
ian farmer obsessed with silkworms. In 1807, when his eyesight
had failed him, Bassi left his job as a lawyer and returned to Lodi,
the farming village where he'd grown up. Trained in science as well
as law, Bassi wrote a series of books and articles on an array of top-
ics, from shepherding to cultivating potatoes to making cheese and
wine.

Bassi was obsessed with one puzzle, however, that would con-
sume him for decades. The country's silkworms were dying from a
disease called *calcinaccio,* or muscardine. The cause was unknown,
and Bassi would launch a nearly twenty-five-year study to figure
it out.

His persistence paid off. In the second decade of investigation,
Bassi noted a white efflorescence had attached itself to the sick
worms. He turned his focus to this intruder, which he would identify as a fungus. He found that the fungus was spreading on dead
worms, and when he transferred it to healthy worms, they would
fall terminally ill. The fungus was a pathogen, and contagious—a
heretical conclusion at a time when doctors and scientists believed
the miasma theory of disease, the idea that noxious vapors caused
illness.

Bassi announced his findings in 1834 at the University of Pavia in front of a crowd of silkworm cultivators. To battle the contamination, he stressed the importance of sterilization, worker hygiene, and minimum exposure to germs. (In the 1860s the French microbiologist Louis Pasteur would cite Bassi in his monumental work on germ theory, as he and German scientist Robert Koch normalized the idea that microorganisms called pathogens caused many human diseases.)

At the turn of the twentieth century, most doctors did not regularly consider fungi when treating sick patients. This started to change in the United States in the 1890s, when Dr. Caspar Gilchrist, who would join the Johns Hopkins bacteriological research laboratory, examined two men from California's Central Valley who died from what appeared to be tuberculosis, a bacterial disease. Both men, Portuguese immigrants who'd worked on farms, had been in agony from an infection that caused "horribly destructive" lesions throughout their body and organs. But tests for the bacterium that caused tuberculosis were negative. Instead, Gilchrist would identify the fungus *Coccidioides* as the cause—the first diagnosed cases of Valley fever, a potentially deadly fungal disease that continues to afflict farmworkers and residents of certain areas of California and the Southwestern U.S. to this day.

The field of medical mycology, the study of fungal diseases in humans, grew in popularity as fungal pathogens were implicated in other perplexing cases. Doctors began to be trained for the first time to consider fungi along with bacteria and viruses in their differential diagnoses. The first cases of fungal meningitis in the United States were reported in New York in 1916, and Columbia University College of Physicians and Surgeons would launch the first full-time medical mycology laboratory in the nation a decade later, in 1926. A dogged research scientist named Rhoda Benham oversaw its creation just as women were being allowed to earn doctorates at

Columbia. Her lab would train a generation of scientists, including Elizabeth Hazen, who along with Rachel Fuller Brown developed nystatin, the first effective antifungal drug.

Still, in the 1920s most research into fungal disease revolved around crops. It was in this scientific milieu that Drechsler described what would later be named *Exserohilum rostratum* when, a few years into his job with the Department of Agriculture, he was asked to investigate a major problem afflicting cereal crops. Plant diseases with monstrous names like spot blotch, foot rot, eyespot, net blotch, and stripe were devastating commercial cereal crops like rice and barley around the globe. Each night after dinner with his family, Drechsler settled in at his desk to draw handsome, skilled renderings of dozens of fungal species. His microscope was outfitted with a camera lucida, a contraption with a lens and a mirror held in place by a metal rod. The lucida, when looked through just right, projected the image under his microscope onto a piece of drawing paper. He would trace the outlines of the microbe he saw there, then use a pen and India ink to draw it, dot by dot, in the pointillist style that he'd learned at Harvard. His wife often had to coax him away from his desk at one or two in the morning.

Dreschler focused in particular on *E. rostratum*'s conidia, drawing the chambered reproductive spores at the top of the page, each with its distinct scar. On the right side of his sheet he sketched an overhead view of a conidium that demonstrated the spindly leglike hyphae radiating from it. The scars developed in the spot where the spore disconnected from the hypha, launching out into the world to reproduce.

At the time, few of the world's fungi were known, and each specimen was a revelation. Drechsler's samples of stink grass alone would yield twelve novel fungal species. (A decade later, some fungi in this group would be reclassified under a new genus, named in his honor: *Drechslera*.) There was one he believed to be of the genus *Hel-*

minthosporium, a collection of dematiaceous, or darkly pigmented, fungi. It needed a name that described the elongated, caterpillar-like spores. He settled on the word *rostrate,* a zoological term meaning beak-like. *Helminthosporium rostratum.*

In the 1940s, fungal diseases were ravaging soldiers fighting in

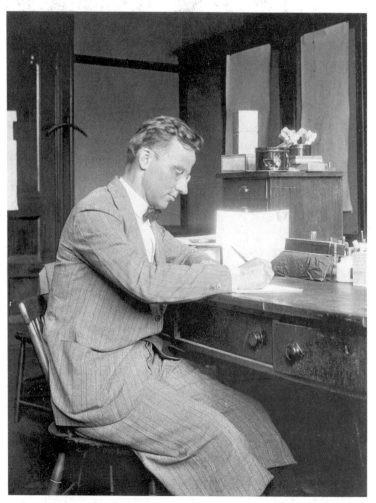

In this undated photo, Charles Drechsler works at his desk while doing post-graduate work at Harvard University. *(Courtesy of the Botany Libraries photograph collection, Harvard University)*

the theaters of Europe, driving Elizabeth Hazen and Rachel Fuller's research into the development of nystatin, the first official antifungal medication. In 1955, researchers extracted amphotericin B from a bacterium found on the banks of the Orinoco River in Venezuela. For decades those two drugs were our best weapons against a broad spectrum of fungi, but amphotericin B could also cause organ failure or other fatal complications in patients. It wasn't until AIDS began to decimate a generation in the eighties and nineties that another option emerged. AIDS-weakened patients became a new population that opportunistic fungal pathogens could infect. Voriconazole was discovered in the 1980s. But as the AIDS emergency faded in the United States, so, too, did antifungal drug development.

Nearly a century after Dreschler first named *E. rostratum*, doctors still had precious few options to defeat it.

*E*xserohilum rostratum has a spotty biography. After Drechsler named his gnarled, scarred fungus, it largely disappeared from published works until the 1970s, when plant pathologists Kurt Leonard and Edna Suggs found it on some corn leaves. The microbe was somewhat unusual in that it did not attack its host indiscriminately, but moved in only under the right conditions, feeding on dead leaf tissue already damaged by insects.

There was something else about the fungus that surprised Leonard and Suggs: it was a supercharged reproducer. In two days in the lab, one spore had covered a leaf with a carpet of fungal growth. Compared to its biological relatives, it was moving at light speed. Not only that, its spores were able to launch into the air using an electromagnetic mechanism that he had only ever seen in fungi classified as ascomycetes.

But the scars were its hallmark. Leonard and Suggs wanted a

word that captured this trait, and fused the Latin *exsertus*, which means "to thrust out," and *hilum*, the term for a scar left on a seed, to form *Exserohilum*. For varietals with the beak-like, stretched-out spores, or conidia, they'd keep Drechsler's description, *rostratum*. *Exserohilum rostratum*.

Nearly four decades later, sitting at her microscope in a dimly lit lab in Virginia, Beverly Jones and her colleagues would recognize it in the spinal fluid of a patient who had died from fungal meningitis. While she had been able to track down a decent amount of information about *E. rostratum*'s pathogenic relationship with plants, it appeared that no one had ever studied its ability to adapt to a human's central nervous system.

The temperature of a healthy human body is 37 degrees Celsius (98.6 degrees Fahrenheit). This warmth serves an important immune function, neutralizing many intruders before they can get comfortable. About three hundred fungal pathogens, like the one behind the white-nose syndrome wiping out the world's population of bats, can grow at 37 degrees and cause disease in humans and other mammals.

For *Exserohilum rostratum* to gain purchase in a human host, it needed a lot of help. The fungus is commonly found in grasses and soil, and it thrives in humid climates, including in NECC's home state of Massachusetts. Healthy people inhale it regularly with few problems; human skin and cilia are among our first-line defenses. If NECC's contaminated steroids had been administered orally, the most common drug delivery method until the mid-1920s, the fungus would have perished in stomach acid. The move toward delivering drugs by injection opened a new pathway into the human body. The invention of disposable plastic syringes in 1955 increased the speed and ubiquity of the method—no more cleaning and re-loading needles, as in the old days. In 1926, the U.S. Pharmaco-peia, the pharmacy industry's safety standards setter and creator of the country's official drug "cookbook," for the first time listed two injectable medications. By 2013, the USP listed 566 different types of approved drug injections. For an opportunist like *E. rostratum,* this innovation was its Trojan horse.

The fungus also needed food and a suitable environment in which to germinate. And it had competition. Scientists at the FDA and the CDC found bacteria and other species of fungi, including molds from the genera *Cladosporium* and *Aspergillus,* in NECC's drugs. But at 37 degrees Celsius in a CDC lab, *E. rostratum* out-competed the others.

Next, *E. rostratum,* previously known to eat only dead plant tis-sue, developed a taste for blood. Doctors at the CDC suspected that it was drawn in by the iron, which is also found in the leaves of plants.

E. rostratum also had help fighting the immune systems of its hosts—the steroid itself. Inflammation, the cause of the back pain in most of the outbreak patients, is a normal immune response, an alarm that sounds in the presence of a pathogen or injury. When a pathogen invades, the immune system calls in its soldiers, white blood cells like T cells, B cells, monocytes, and granulocytes like neutrophils. Steroids suppress this immune response, reducing in-flammation and its accompanying pain, and buying *E. rostratum* time to grow and multiply.

E. rostratum had another advantage: pigmentation. Dematia-ceous molds, so-called because of the brown and black melanin in their cell walls, are able to gird themselves against another human defense. When a pathogen invades, the immune system triggers bursts of oxygen and nitrogen to neutralize it, but some pigmented fungal pathogens react to oxidative burst attacks by adapting their DNA. Instead of dying, the molds learn to withstand it.

With such good fortune, *E. rostratum* thrived. So why would it kill such an amenable host?

There is a stark difference between fungi and other pathogens, like bacteria. In his book about the cholera epidemic in nineteenth-century London, *The Ghost Map*, Steven Johnson explains: "A lethal strain can make untold billions of copies of itself in a matter of hours, but that reproductive success usually kills off the human body that made that reproduction possible. If those billion copies don't find their way into another intestinal tract quickly, the whole process is for naught." A bacterial pathogen like *Vibrio cholerae* sometimes will slow its reproduction down to keep its host alive. But fungi don't need a live host to survive. In fact, most feed on dead tissue.

"When [fungal pathogens] get into an ecosystem—a vertebrate host, for example—they simply don't care," said molecular microbiologist and immunologist Dr. Arturo Casadevall in *Fungal Diseases: An Emerging Threat to Human, Animal, and Plant Health*, a workshop and report funded by the National Institutes of Health in 2011. "They have no need for that host in order to go forward. They will take down every last member of the species." For invading fungi, the host's death is part of the equation.

CHAPTER 10

THE CASE OF A CAREER

OCTOBER 2012

THE U.S. ATTORNEY'S OFFICE, WASHINGTON, D.C.

George Varghese typed "fungal meningitis" into his browser, the receiver for his desk phone scrunched between his shoulder and his ear. From his office on the eleventh floor of the U.S. attorney's building in Washington, D.C., he could see the Capitol's dome in the distance. On the line was Jack Pirozzolo, the second-in-command at the U.S. Attorney's Office in Boston, which prosecutes federal crimes in Massachusetts. "You probably know about the fungal meningitis outbreak?" Jack was asking.

"Sure I do," Varghese lied. He clicked through the links as Pirozzolo talked, his eyes darting through headlines about the rising death toll.

"Look, we don't know if there's a crime here, but we want you to investigate it," Pirozzolo said.

As a federal prosecutor for seven years, Varghese had distinguished himself in the terrorism unit of the DOJ. When Pirozzolo called, Varghese was working a case that would make headlines: a man named Oscar Ortega-Hernandez had fired ten gunshots at the White House.

The hard-charging culture of Washington was a good fit for Varghese, a former Wall Street investment banker who had grown up in Potomac, the son of Indian immigrants. But his wife had always wanted to move back to New England, so he had recently interviewed for a job in the U.S. Attorney's Office in Boston, which had a reputation for taking on health care fraud and organized crime, most notably James "Whitey" Bulger and Francis "Cadillac Frank" Salemme, head of the New England Cosa Nostra. Instead of going after mobsters, though, the office wanted Varghese to join its health care fraud unit, which needed someone with his trial experience. NECC was not yet on anyone's radar and the move did not seem a good fit for his ambition. He pictured going after Medicare fraud and medical device executives, white-collar cases in Boston that would be cordial, sleepy affairs compared to fighting terrorism in the nation's capital. Plus, he'd have to master a whole new area of law.

But as he skimmed the headlines Varghese saw that dozens of people in multiple states were victims of contaminated drugs. It was high profile and would be complicated. He understood little about compounding pharmacies, let alone the web of federal laws that govern manufacturing drugs. Varghese would have to talk to doctors, mycologists, anesthesiologists, epidemiologists. *Aspergillus fumigatus, Exserohilum rostratum.* The U.S. Pharmacopeia. Suddenly the health care unit looked more exciting.

As thousands of terrified patients rushed to hospitals in Tennessee, Michigan, Indiana, Virginia, Florida, and North Carolina, his family packed the car and drove north.

THE U.S. ATTORNEY'S OFFICE, BOSTON

Amanda Strachan stood in her office, her heart racing. Her boss was considering giving away the biggest case she'd ever seen, and she wanted to stop him. Strachan was not good at masking her emotions. As a federal health care fraud prosecutor, she was obsessed with the fungal meningitis crisis. She refreshed CNN's website every few hours to check the ever-rising death toll, released regularly by the CDC. The largest drug contamination outbreak in modern U.S. history was unfolding in her backyard, and she was at risk of losing the opportunity to prosecute it before it even began. But not without a fight.

Earlier that year, the health care fraud unit had faced a devastating public embarrassment that was the talk of the Boston legal community for weeks. After a years-long fraud investigation into the president of a medical device maker, Stryker Biotech Corporation, the government had been forced to settle the case. Its star witnesses—the doctors who were scheduled to speak out about being defrauded by Stryker—had recanted and agreed to testify for the defense. Strachan's colleagues had failed to properly interview and vet the doctors, and Stryker's defense team pounced. U.S. attorney Carmen Ortiz, head honcho of the Massachusetts district office, issued a statement afterward saying there had been a "strategic error in preparing for trial."

Strachan, who was not involved in the Stryker case, was one of only a handful of attorneys remaining in the unit after a shake-up. A veteran Massachusetts state homicide prosecutor, Nathaniel "Nat" Yeager, had been brought in to lead the rebuilt group. He had been there only a few months when NECC became the office's top case. Given the recent upheaval, the U.S. attorney, Ortiz, was leaning toward assigning the investigation to a more senior prosecutor in the drug or public corruption units. Strachan sensed that Yeager was also forming the opinion that the health care unit was not up to the task.

As a mother of three boys, Strachan was always prepared, armed with plastic action figures in her purse to pull out whenever her kids got restless. But now she was acting on pure passion. "If you send this case out of the unit you are telling the world that we can't do this, and we *can* do it," she argued. Yeager agreed to keep the nascent probe in the group, but his concerns hung like a fog over the investigation.

Strachan's specialty was companies who committed Medicare fraud, as well as off-label production of drugs. NECC was a much more complicated case, with victims spread around the country. But she felt instinctually that she was the one to do it. She had grown up in Needham, a middle-class Boston suburb close to Framingham, where NECC was based, and attended Boston University Law School. These people—the pharmacy's owners and employees—were her neighbors.

Yeager assigned Strachan to manage the discovery phase leading up to the trial, investigating and collecting evidence. Autopsy reports. Medical files. Emails. Phone records. Hospital drug order forms. Initially she felt honored to be given a crucial, but thankless, role in such a mammoth case. She also felt a burning desire to prove herself. Soon she was battling a growing sense of disappointment about being given what she considered an administrative job, while four male prosecutors took on more visible positions. Even so, it would probably be the most important case on which she'd ever work.

Strachan's first task was to answer a key question: Who were the victims? Media reported that the CDC was tracking the toll, so she called the headquarters in Atlanta to request a list of names. She was quickly shut down. In determining the scope of the epidemic, the CDC was concerned with population-level data—the number of infected people, their locations, and their symptoms. From their standpoint, a patient's identity went no farther than the state and the case number. The state public health departments also refused to hand over the information, citing laws that protect patient privacy.

When Strachan told them that the federal patient privacy law, the HIPAA Privacy Rule, had an exemption for law enforcement, they still didn't budge. She'd have to get a subpoena.

As Strachan dug in, an unfamiliar face joined the team: George Varghese. She thought he had the air of the "anointed one" in from Washington with the blessings of the higher levels of the Department of Justice. But interoffice politics did not faze him. He had joined the health care unit with a clear mandate: to lead the NECC investigation. Its success and his were intertwined. When he arrived for his first day, four attorneys, including Yeager and Strachan, were already deep into their research. Each investigator was operating independently, filing subpoenas and interviewing witnesses without the others' knowledge. For a case with hundreds of witnesses and millions of company records, Varghese felt like it was chaos.

Strachan shared Varghese's unhappiness with the lack of direction. She may have had the least amount of visible responsibility, but he thought she was the most promising attorney on the case. He understood little about health care law, and her expertise was clear. When he sent out emails to the team with updated findings about NECC, she was often the only one who responded.

Varghese had the backing of the DOJ, and Strachan could maneuver the personalities in Boston. They made a pact. They would conduct every interview in tandem. They would negotiate offers to witnesses together. Subpoenas. All of it. They would take the case over by mastering its complexities together.

Strachan's background in medical fraud influenced her thinking about the crimes she could charge against Barry Cadden and NECC. It was a clear-cut case of fraud, she thought. About two months into the investigation, Fred Wyshak, her colleague in Boston, offered an alternative. Wyshak, one of the country's top organized crime prosecutors, told her: "That's a RICO murder case," using a shorthand term for the federal racketeering laws he had used to prosecute Bulger and Salemme. Strachan smiled and thought: "Fred, you see RICO when you buy coffee in the morning." She dismissed the comment as a wry quip from a veteran mob prosecutor. These were pharmacists, not mobsters.

MILLIS, MASSACHUSETTS

Owen Finnegan endured a constant knot of anxiety since the production line had been shut down. Human Resources sent a few emails saying that NECC, which had now recalled all of its products, still hoped to reopen. Finnegan knew the emails were bullshit. Dozens of people had died, and hundreds more had contracted meningitis from the vials that he had filled. Was it his fault? The thoughts plagued his sleep, and his feelings of guilt threatened his already shaky marriage. In the meantime, he had no job and was living on unemployment.

A lawyer hired by the NECC called Finnegan. The company was happy to provide its former employees with free legal counsel, he was told, and some of his coworkers had already taken the offer. But Finnegan was aware that the company would ultimately protect its own interests above all. He kept obsessing on the conversation he'd had with pharmacist Gene Svirskiy just before that day when they'd all been told to go home. Svirskiy had warned Finnegan to prepare for questions from the inspectors. Finnegan could easily be the fall guy. And now they wanted to provide him with an attorney? *What benefit does NECC get from paying for my lawyer other than to keep me quiet about what happened?* he thought.

His family contacted the one legal expert they trusted: Dennis Brown, an attorney for the Wellesley Fire Department's union, where Finnegan's uncle was fire chief. Dennis quickly zeroed in on a particular detail of Finnegan's job description. A pharmacist was supposed to double-check Finnegan's work, from filling vials and crimping lids to shipping trays of medicine. Glenn Chin had allowed Finnegan to cut corners, often signing off on his efforts with little more than a glance, to get orders out faster. Brown thought Finnegan would be valuable to prosecutors. He saw an opening for a preemptive strike.

Finnegan initially resisted. There was no guarantee that he would be granted immunity or any benefit from going to the feds. Also, these were his coworkers, some of them close friends. "If you answer their questions truthfully, is it really snitching?" Brown asked. Finally Finnegan agreed to simply lay out the facts. Brown set up a meeting with the U.S. attorney.

Brown was not a member of the tight-knit community of white-collar health care defense lawyers in Boston. Strachan knew them all on a first-name basis, a collegiality useful for making deals. She was used to gamesmanship; defense attorneys always sought assurances that a deal could be struck for their client's testimony. But Brown did not play any games. He said his client just wanted to come in and tell the truth. There were no other terms. Finnegan would answer all of the prosecutors' questions.

The next morning, as Finnegan walked over the rusty bridge spanning the canal to the U.S. Attorney's Office, he thought, *How the fuck did I get in this position?* A few months earlier he'd had the best job of his life, buddies at work, and a happy bride. Now his job was in tatters, he was afraid he might face prison time, his marriage was under strain, and his colleagues had started to turn against one another.

He and Brown sat across from federal prosecutors in a conference room with windows that looked out over Boston Harbor. Two FDA agents were at the end of the table. If Finnegan's story held up, he might escape prosecution, but there were no promises.

Finnegan barely took a breath as he spoke. It was early in the
investigation, and federal prosecutors still did not understand how
NECC worked. Over the course of several weeks, Finnegan would
meet with prosecutors many times, and explain it all: Chin made
the methylpred, and Finnegan filled the mixed drug into individual vials that were then shipped to customers. He outlined how the
pharmacists regularly mixed expired batches of drugs with newer
lots to deceive customers. When a chemical was beyond reuse, the
techs would flush it down the sink into the city sewer system. Employees regularly forged cleaning logs to make it look as if they'd
scrubbed their workstations when they hadn't. There were flies and
bugs in the clean room, and tumbleweeds of human hair.

Sometimes the petri dishes that NECC used to test for contaminants showed mold hits. Varghese stopped Finnegan. What? Finnegan repeated himself: the company's environmental monitor,
Annette Robinson, tested regularly for mold, and numerous times
in 2012, those tests came back positive.

Oh my God, Varghese thought. Dozens of people had died so far,
and it wasn't due to an accident. There was a long-term pattern
emerging. To him, NECC sounded like a criminal enterprise.

In December, less than three months since the start of the outbreak, a federal judge empaneled a criminal grand jury, a secret
proceeding where a group of citizens are chosen at random to hear
evidence. There is no judge or defense to cross-examine anyone.
This was where Varghese and Strachan would begin to build their
case, witness by witness. At the end, when the prosecutors rest a
case, the jury can issue an indictment or decide the prosecution has
not demonstrated probable cause. Finnegan would be among the
first NECC employees called to testify.

Word got around that the U.S. Attorney's Office had obtained a
formidable amount of information about the compounder's internal
workings. When confronted by Varghese and Strachan, other phar-

macy techs, who initially said they had not seen anything suspicious, changed their tune. Glenn Chin's personal technician, Corey Fletcher, the man who made the methylpred alongside him, eventually cooperated, too. Strachan and Varghese's bosses said they wanted an indictment within two years. The clock was ticking.

CHAPTER 11

THE HAIL MARY

OCTOBER 2012

BARRINGTON, ILLINOIS

Sarah Sellers's long-haired German shepherd sat at her feet. Sunlight warmed her home office as she settled into another workday with a cup of coffee. Five years earlier, she had left the FDA and pushed the compounding pharmacy issue to the background in her life. Her divorce was behind her and she was getting paid well doing drug safety work for manufacturers, living happily with her kids in suburban Chicago.

Her phone rang. It was a friend, an infectious disease doctor. "There's an unbelievable situation unfolding in Tennessee related to a compounded drug," he said. His brother, an anesthesiologist at the St. Thomas Medical Center in Nashville, was on the front lines of the first wave of infected patients.

As he spoke, Sellers's peaceful life faded away, and she felt hollow. Nearly a decade earlier, she had warned the Senate about the public health dangers of compounded injectable drugs. Now dozens of people were fighting off a killer fungus. This was the Big One that she had known would come sooner or later. A CNN reporter called and asked to do a story about her prior work.

Within days an email from an old colleague at the FDA popped into her inbox; it would bring Sellers back into the fold. "A number of us would like to catch up on your latest wisdom about the facts, policies, and politics of compounding," it read. The agency saw the outbreak as an opportunity to reform the law and wanted her help. Policy advisers working on Capitol Hill started calling, too, seeking her counsel on the updated rules that Congress should draft.

She felt the old pull to help, and would jump back into the fray. This was the chance for the country to find a real solution to the compounding problem. The process would be full of twists and turns, she knew, but it was worth a shot.

DAY 58, NOVEMBER 14, 2012: 32 DEAD, MORE THAN 400 CASES

WASHINGTON, D.C.

Joyce Lovelace faced the row of stern-faced lawmakers on the House Energy and Commerce Committee, which oversees the FDA. The legislators peered down at her from a dais in the resonant, high-ceilinged hearing room. It was November 14, 2012. Over the past weeks her husband had died of an unknown disease and was buried, and then exhumed and autopsied. The autopsy had confirmed that he was a victim of the fungus *Exserohilum rostratum*. Now Joyce was resolute and ready to tell her husband's story, the only victim scheduled to testify. She had no notes. Judge Eddie didn't believe in reading in front of people, so she would speak from the heart, like he would have.

It had been nearly two months since the first cases of the outbreak were revealed in Tennessee. The microbe's grisly march was on the wane. But confusion and bitterness remained. How could thousands of people have been exposed to contaminated drugs here in the United States? Now legislators, especially in the affected states, were paying attention.

Joyce was the first witness in a series of investigative hearings that would stretch on for months to look into the gaps in oversight and other failures that led to the outbreak. Perhaps a compounding pharmacy safety law would give meaning to her otherwise pointless loss. She sat with her hands folded as she listened to the committee members' opening statements.

Speaking in a Kentucky twang, Joyce described the nightmare she had just lived through. "People, it was not an easy death that we witnessed," she said with slow seriousness, describing Judge Eddie's rapid decline. She paused. "Whoever is responsible, I want them to know that their lack of attention to their duties cost my husband his life. Cost my family.

"I cannot beg you enough. Bipartisan, I don't care what party. Work together so that no family will have to go through what we have."

The GOP-controlled committee would produce an inflammatory forty-three-page investigative report titled *FDA's Oversight of NECC and Ameridose: A History of Missed Opportunities?* It outlined the times, from 2002 to 2011, that the FDA had received complaints from Colorado and other state pharmacy officials about NECC and its sister company Ameridose, including concerns over the safety of its drugs. The paper blamed the agency's paralysis over its legal authority for not acting more assertively to shut NECC down before it was too late. These criticisms—drafted with the help of the industry's lobbying group, the International Academy of Compounding Pharmacists—pointed the finger back at the Obama administration's FDA commissioner, Margaret Hamburg, who was leading the charge on updated regulations for compounders.

The committee's report concluded: "Additional authority will not necessarily solve the fundamental issues within FDA that allowed this tragedy to unfold right under the agency's nose."

Hamburg, a Harvard Medical School graduate and career bureaucrat who had been at the FDA for only a few years, had little knowledge of compounding policy. She had been briefed by staff and FDA attorneys, but had not mastered the law's complexities when she appeared to testify before the committee. She did have a warning to share, though. "There's thousands of other compounders out there . . . and thus many other firms with the potential to generate a tragedy like this," she told the lawmakers. "We need these compounders of high risk products to register with us. We need inspectional authority and full access to records . . . and clearly there should be a uniform set of standards for safety practices and quality manufacturing."

Republican congresswoman Marsha Blackburn of Tennessee and others kept the hearing focused on the FDA's contribution in the disaster. If the agency had been so ineffective, they argued, it was undeserving of an increase in its oversight powers. A few months earlier, Congresswoman Blackburn accepted a $10,000 donation from the IACP. Now she wanted to know if the FDA had ever responded to a complaint from the state of Colorado's pharmacy board about NECC's selling drugs without valid prescriptions.

"Did you even pick up the telephone and call the Massachusetts board of pharmacy and say, 'We think we have a repeat offender?'" Blackburn asked, pointing her finger at Hamburg.

"I understand what you're getting at there, but . . ." Hamburg said quietly.

"Yes or no, did you pick up the phone and call?" Blackburn interrupted.

"Email was being used," Hamburg replied.

"Would you like to supply all of those emails to us for the record?" Blackburn shot back.

"I believe you have them," Hamburg said.

Republican representative Joe Barton of Texas, who had accepted $7,500 from IACP prior to the hearing, pivoted the conversation to accuse the FDA commissioner of opportunism. "Apparently the FDA has decided this is something that they can use to be able to get more authority to inspect certain transactions that compounding pharmacies do," he said indignantly. The IACP had warned its members to watch out for overreach in the days leading up to the hearing.

Hamburg was unable to explain the agency's inaction to their liking, saying only that the FDA tried to use its authority, but only in reaction to problems that rose to their attention.

Republican representative Morgan Griffith, whose Virginia district included hundreds of people who had been exposed to NECC's tainted steroids, and who would become a regular recipient of thousands of dollars in donations from the IACP, also criticized Hamburg's request for more authority.

"It's very frustrating when you come in here and say [the FDA's] authority wasn't clear. These folks were manufacturing, what are you doing now to find out if there's somebody else out there?" Griffith said, confusing the role of the FDA to oversee manufacturers with the role of the state to regulate pharmacies.

"Your question speaks directly to why do we need legislation and new authorities. Compounding pharmacies are not required—" Hamburg said.

"Hang on." Griffith cut her off. "I'm telling you from the evidence I heard today it appears these were manufacturers. You keep going back to compounding and that's why everybody's getting frustrated with you," he said, again asserting the idea that NECC was manufacturing illegally by exploiting a loophole in the law and registering as a pharmacy.

"I think we really do need to clarify that in legislation in terms of—" Hamburg responded.

"I already heard that," Griffith said, a measure of disgust in his voice as he cut her off.

After listening to hours of combative testimony, Michigan representative John Dingell had heard enough. A veteran Democrat in his eighties with a deep understanding of drug policy, he represented a state with 129 confirmed cases and nine deaths, the most in the nation. "It appears that New England Compounding Center, and other like-hearted rascals, have engaged in the practice of figuring themselves a fine loophole in which through lobbying and other efforts they have been able to ensure that they're able to engage in practices that impose substantial dangers on the American people."

The hearing ended without a clear resolution. The Democratic members who were seeking greater oversight authority for the FDA over compounders had been stymied by their colleagues who blamed the agency.

Joyce Lovelace still harbored hope that some measure of legal protection could be achieved. She sent the committee a letter urging them to come together to prevent another tragedy. "Put aside partisan politics, partisan philosophies, industry lobbying, and wishes of campaign contributions and unanimously send to the White House a bill that will prevent a recurrence of these events," Lovelace pleaded.

"If you will do that, perhaps my family can take some solace in the fact that Eddie Lovelace's public service continues even after death."

Instead, Congressman Griffith sponsored a House bill the following year to deny the FDA any added authority. The draft cemented the status quo: the FDA would still have to ask states for permission before going into a compounding pharmacy for an inspection, and compounders were allowed to mix large batches of drugs without prescriptions. The bill also permitted hospitals to send lists of patient names after the fact—"backfilling" orders, just as NECC had done. The bill fulfilled most of the IACP's wildest dreams.

When Sarah Sellers read early versions of Griffith's bill, she was perplexed. From her office in suburban Chicago, she'd worked for weeks with congressional staffers to guide them through the complicated world of pharmacy compounding law, but the language in front of her maintained the piecemeal system that had allowed NECC to operate free of oversight and actually *eroded* the FDA's ability to hold bad actors to account.

But there was still hope. Developing and passing legislation is a marathon process. A different bill would take form on the other side of the Capitol in the Senate.

THE NEXT DAY

U.S. SENATE COMMITTEE ON HEALTH, EDUCATION, LABOR, AND PENSIONS

"All of us are shaken," said Senator Lamar Alexander of Tennessee. "We live in this country where we have this miracle that we walk into one of our sixty-thousand drugstores or pharmacies, or go to our doctor or pain clinic, and we don't think about it. We just assume it's safe."

Alexander spoke into a microphone to his colleagues in the old library-like room that houses the Senate's Health, Education, Labor and Pensions (HELP) Committee. A day after the House's hearing, the committee had called FDA commissioner Hamburg as well as the head lobbyist of the IACP to testify. The atmosphere was less tense in the Democratic-controlled Senate, even as Republicans like Alexander spoke.

"Whose job will it be to make sure it doesn't happen again?" he asked. It was time to put someone "on the flagpole." He explained, "As governor sometimes I gave jobs to multiple people and it wouldn't get done. But if I gave it to one person, I put somebody on the flagpole, it was amazing to see that responsibility got done. Let's put the state pharmacy [boards] on the flagpole or the FDA on the flagpole and let's get the other out of it."

David Miller, IACP's executive vice president and CEO, listened as lawmaker after lawmaker called for stronger oversight of his industry, a profound pivot from the hearing on the day before over in the GOP-led House. His group had fought off regulation for years. The IACP was now organizing its most forceful effort in its twenty-year history.

The stakes for the IACP and its burgeoning industry had never been higher. Even conservative states-rights senators like Alexander were pushing for tougher regulations. Miller's goal, as it had been the day before, was to undermine the FDA's credibility and thus their request for more control. Few lawmakers made any effort to understand the FDA's history of attempts to gain legal oversight of compounders, rendering the agency an easy scapegoat.

"Ultimately, how do we assure that compounding pharmacists are able to practice their professional expertise without overly burdensome regulations?" Miller said in his opening remarks. "Something we find particularly disturbing is that the agency who knew that NECC was distributing drugs without patient-specific prescriptions throughout the United States did *nothing* to stop them."

HELP Committee chair Democratic Iowa senator Tom Harkin was alarmed to learn about the lack of a watchdog, which meant the federal government had failed to stop NECC before it was too late. But the Senate committee believed that the FDA needed to be given the legal authority Hamburg sought to stop another disaster. Even Harkin's Republican colleagues had started to see things this way, due in large part to Senator Pat Roberts, still the most knowledgeable lawmaker in Washington on the compounding issue. Roberts's key staffer on the bill was a senior health policy adviser, Jennifer Boyer, who had realized there was ambiguity in the law that had created a gaping loophole when it came to oversight. "Everything didn't work, that was the problem," Boyer explained after reading hundreds of pages of compounding policy background she'd requested from the Congressional Research Service. "You go to the state level, and they say, 'We can only go into a compounding pharmacy once every three years.' Then FDA says, 'We can't get access to the bad actors, and when we do they sue and their records disappear.'"

The FDA had been ineffective, there was no question about that. But it was also true that the agency did not have authority over compounders as it did over drug manufacturers. As Hamburg had testified, the FDA could react to problems at compounders only after people were sick and dying. Its inspectors could enter pharmacies only with prior permission or a subpoena—and businesses with something to hide always demanded a subpoena, removing the element of surprise.

The Senate's draft bill that would take form in the coming months, unlike the House bill, granted most of the FDA's wishes. It created a framework to help the FDA detect and respond to businesses like NECC, including requiring regular federal inspections of all compounding pharmacies. It also proposed a new regulatory category called "compound manufacturers" that would encompass any pharmacy that made large quantities of sterile drugs and shipped them across state lines. The public also needed data: how many compounders were there, and how many drugs did they make? The Senate's draft bill mandated reporting of patient harm so that the FDA could better keep track.

Reading versions of the Senate draft from Chicago, Sellers thought it was a step in the right direction. After numerous legislative failures, perhaps this one would finally make it through.

DAY 286, JULY 1, 2013: 61 DEAD, 749 CASES

Ten months had passed since Tom Rybinski arrived at the ER as patient zero. By the time the Senate's bill was drafted, the CDC had already ceased regular tracking of the death toll. Marion Kainer, Ben Park, Rachel Smith and their colleagues, as well as state health departments and clinics, had confirmed that the contaminated vials were out of harm's way. The public health system had limited the damage, identifying *Exserohilum rostratum* and likely saving many lives by removing the contaminated steroids from circulation and aggressively treating patients with antifungals.

Now the pressure was on Congress to fix the law.

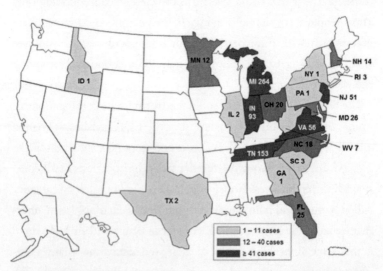

A map of fungal meningitis cases produced by the CDC during the 2012–2013 outbreak. *(Courtesy of the U.S. Centers for Disease Control and Prevention)*

The Senate signaled it was ready for an early vote on its version of the bill. Senator Alexander would accept donations from the IACP, but the relationship had soured to the point that the lobbying group had stopped returning his staffer's calls. The compounding group's CEO, David Miller, took emergency action.

Hundreds of compounding pharmacists arrived in Washington from all over the country. "We have very critical issues before us as a profession. Perhaps like never before," the IACP's latest policy update had read. It would be a scorched-earth effort: for any pharmacists who couldn't storm Capitol Hill in person, the group organized an online campaign to spam lawmakers. "With IACP's Virtual Hill Day, you can still make a real difference."

They marched down the echoey hallways of Capitol Hill and by the dozens buttonholed their representatives. The Senate bill would destroy small businesses in their districts, they argued. Regulations would only *hurt* patients by depriving them of important compounded medications, they explained. There was little pushback from the other side. Many of the fungal meningitis patients who had survived were still sick or preoccupied with reassembling lives disrupted by illness. Most Americans still didn't even know what a compounding pharmacy was. After the initial sensational headlines, the story had dropped from the front pages altogether. This vacuum, plus a million dollars in lobbying efforts—more than the previous four years combined—acted as a megaphone to amplify IACP's voice.

The industry's message once again resonated with some members of Congress, especially in the "Compounding Belt" states of Florida, Georgia, Louisiana, and Alabama.

"Unfortunately, the same folks that were active to prohibit our efforts to address the compounding issue in 2002 and 2007, they're back at it again," Senator Roberts said when addressing a second

HELP Committee hearing in May 2013 as the Senate worked to finalize its bill. "I want everyone listening, everyone here in this committee room . . . to know that our legislation does not prohibit access to lifesaving medication and therapies for patients."

As David Miller looked on from the sidelines, Senator Roberts joked, "The penalty for not understanding this will be to go to Dodge City, where you will be hung by the neck until you are dead."

Roberts's tough talk would not cow the IACP. It began targeting staff members working on the bill, including his main health policy analyst, Jennifer Boyer. One blog post on the website of an IACP-affiliated group called the Alliance for Natural Health read "Drug Companies Plan to Use Compounding Bill to Take Away Your Compounded Medications." The post suggested that Boyer was a Big Pharma industry plant trying to get rid of the competition at the behest of her husband, Dave Boyer, who worked as a lobbyist for BGR Group, which represents both pharmaceutical and pharmacy industry clients. "If you think this sounds like a conflict of interest, you're right: in meetings she has been a strident voice against compounding."

Mailers started to circulate calling for Senator Roberts to fire Boyer, and she received harassing phone calls at work: "We know who you are. We know who your husband works for." Her office began screening her telephone calls. Compounding pharmacists in his state argued for her ouster to the senator in person. But he refused.

SEPTEMBER 2013

Congress was stalled. The Senate's bipartisan coalition supported giving the FDA the powers it needed to oversee drug compounders, while the House, led by Republican Morgan Griffith, refused.

Competing House and Senate bills stood in conflict. Neither side would budge.

After months of negotiation, the FDA policy advisers for the Senate HELP Committee believed it was time to walk away. If Griffith's law passed, they believed it would actually impair public safety. President Obama had gone through a bruising, years-long fight with Congress over the Affordable Care Act and there was little will within the administration for another protracted health care battle.

Elizabeth Jungman, who worked for the Senate committee's chair, Harkin, was feeling particularly frustrated when she arrived to give a speech at a hospital pharmacy lobby's annual breakfast. The group had split with the IACP to support the Senate bill. Now she had to deliver a disappointment: the negotiations were in jeopardy. The pharmacists told her to keep pushing. Hospitals needed safe compounded drugs, and they were terrified of another outbreak.

Jungman emerged from the breakfast reenergized. Within the vacuum of Capitol Hill, it was easy to lose sight of what was really at stake—patients' lives. Congress was on the precipice of doing something. But the Senate could not pass their version all alone.

If House Republicans would not agree to mandated federal supervision of compounding pharmacies, what about a voluntary option? Jungman proposed adding Section 503B to the Food, Drug, and Cosmetic Act to allow owners of larger pharmacies, like Barry Cadden, to *choose* FDA scrutiny (which they already could). But this new section offered an additional carrot. Compounders that endured FDA oversight would be rewarded with the right to make more drugs without prescriptions from a list of FDA-approved, bulk active pharmaceutical ingredients. The actual list was to be negotiated later. Traditional pharmacies would remain covered under the existing law, 503A, and states would still oversee this vast majority of compounders.

It would not change the situation much, but might make everyone a little safer by giving hospitals a list of compounders that volunteered for oversight and used FDA-approved ingredients. The idea quickly gained support in both chambers, still under public pressure to respond to the NECC tragedy.

When Sarah Sellers received the updated legislation for review, though, she felt dismayed once again at its imperfections. The FDA had asked Congress for legal clarity. This bill only complicated things further by creating two systems: the state-led status quo that exempted most compounding pharmacies from the Food, Drug, and Cosmetic Act, and a voluntary rule that pharmacy owners like Cadden would never choose to implement.

The Drug Quality and Security Act (DQSA) sailed through both chambers of Congress. On November 27, 2013—about two months after Jungman's Hail Mary saved the negotiations from collapsing altogether—President Barack Obama signed it into law.

At the very least, FDA commissioner Hamburg had asked Congress to require compounding pharmacies to register with the agency. No data existed on the number of compounding pharmacies. No agency or office tracked the drugs they made. No law would be effective without this data. Yet on these basic points the DQSA failed, and compounding pharmacy data remained largely in the shadows. Instead of putting one agency squarely on "the flagpole," the law as enacted only made things messier.

"We missed a golden opportunity. If we were not going to do it then, when could we do it?" said Jennifer Boyer years later, reflecting on her work.

For Sellers, it was yet another example of the industry's growing influence. Before she could return to her normal life, however, there was one more request to consider. She had been nominated to serve on the FDA compounding advisory committee created by the DQSA. "This is not a good time to lose your voice on compounding," a high-ranking FDA official told her. But within a few weeks, the FDA told her she was not needed.

"The IACP won. They're completely unstoppable," Sellers said recently in an interview at her home outside Chicago.

As a thank-you, Congress sent her a framed copy of the final bill with President Obama's signature. She put it in a closet along with all her other compounding records, closing another chapter in a long and bitter struggle.

ALBANY, KENTUCKY

Joyce Lovelace returned to Albany and the small house with walls covered in family photos. She had to live the rest of her life without her best friend, but her children and grandchildren rallied around her, which eased some of the pain.

She had done her part to try to convince Congress to reform

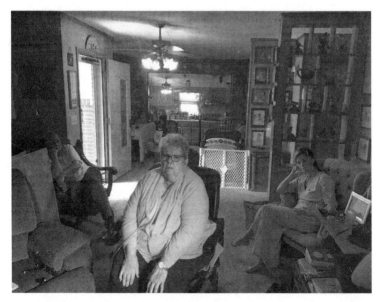

Joyce Lovelace (center), whose husband, Eddie Lovelace, died after being injected with contaminated steroids produced by the New England Compounding Center, sits in her living room in Albany, Kentucky, in 2019. *(Courtesy of the author)*

the industry that killed her husband. When she heard about the passage of the DQSA, she thought some good might come of it. She'd worked in Eddie's law office for decades and was no stranger to the realities of politics. But the more she read about the law, the more disenchanted she became. It seemed that the victims "had been swept under the rug" in Washington's rush to claim a bipartisan success.

There was one more chance for justice, though. Joyce had received a call from federal prosecutors in Boston. Barry Cadden was likely to be criminally charged and arrested, and a trial was on the horizon.

CHAPTER 12

DEPRAVED INDIFFERENCE

2014: 76 DEAD, 778 FUNGAL INFECTIONS

NECC, FRAMINGHAM, MASSACHUSETTS

George Varghese picked up his camera and jumped into the waiting car. More than a year had passed since the start of the NECC investigation. Finally, Varghese and his partner Amanda Strachan were driving a half hour west to NECC headquarters in Framingham to see the clean rooms for themselves. Strachan's subpoenas seeking victim identities had dragged on for months, slowing their collection of evidence to a trickle. But there was still plenty to do with what they had collected from NECC. Investigators had seized some twenty million pages of documents: emails, log formula worksheets, recipes for each batch of drugs, and shipping records. Varghese, Strachan, their paralegal, special agents, and law clerks spent months reading through Glenn Chin's and Barry Cadden's emails, which yielded countless investigative leads.

Months had passed. Then a year. The prosecutors called witnesses to the grand jury nearly every week, slowly building toward a criminal indictment. For now, Cadden and Chin remained out of custody. They pulled into NECC's football-field-sized parking lot and stared at the nondescript brick building. They did not expect to find any new evidence—the FBI, the FDA, pharmacy inspectors, bankruptcy lawyers, and defense attorneys had all picked over it. But they needed to see it for themselves.

As they walked around the main clean room, now grimy after years as a crime scene, Strachan recoiled at the sight of a dead bird on the floor. Varghese snapped pictures. Bottles of chemicals remained on the shelves. The aquarium-like glove boxes stood sentinel. The tables held bottles employees used to spray alcohol on vials of drugs and their workstations. One with an orange sticker marked *Methotrexate* grabbed Varghese's attention: in 2011, there had been a shortage of the chemotherapy drug used for children with leukemia. Varghese recalled an email from Cadden about selling drugs with an active ingredient five years past its usage date. Varghese noted the bottle's expiration date: 2007. Was this the expired batch that they had used to make the chemo drugs that NECC sold to hospitals? He had it bagged and tagged as evidence. He also took photos of the cracks in the floors through which oil still oozed. Chin had had them covered with trash cans during the FBI and Massachusetts pharmacy inspections, so the agents had missed them.

Strachan walked into the second, smaller clean room, where pharmacists made heart-stopping cardioplegia drugs, and picked up a spray bottle that read *Mudgum*. Mudgum was the nickname of a pharmacy tech, Joe Connolly's brother, Scott Connolly, who had lost his license in Massachusetts and had been working at NECC illegally, using Cadden's credentials to log his work.

The prosecutors could not believe what they saw. Within a half hour they had found evidence they could use—expired chemicals, confirmation of an unlicensed worker, and environmental risks.

JUNE 2014

THE ANN ARBOR FEDERAL BUILDING

The soft-spoken, neatly dressed man sat across from Strachan. Kenneth Todd's mother had died after being injected with *Exserohilum rostratum*. A victim witness specialist from the FBI and an FDA agent were in the room, as well as a state prosecutor from the Michigan attorney general's office.

It had taken months and a massive push to get here. After Strachan realized the prosecutors would need to get creative to obtain patient information, they'd set up a shared computer drive known as the Victims Project, which included a massive database of records that they could use to identify the casualties. The CDC simply recorded a number next to the state where a case occurred—*Indiana 94*—so they'd subpoenaed all seventy-six facilities that received contaminated drugs for a list of the patients who'd been given a methylpred shot in the summer of 2012. For the past year, law clerks in the Boston office had cross-referenced the CDC's list of confirmed cases to the clinic records, triangulating the date, location, and drug to assemble the most comprehensive index of the infected: 793 names.

They'd also posted information on the FBI's website, inviting victims to contact them. Now they were sitting down with respondents to find witnesses who could testify before the grand jury. It was the middle of 2014, and they had about six months left before the deadline their boss had set for an indictment.

Strachan was nervous. Health care fraud prosecutors don't usually interview victims' family members. But she'd spent months learning about the conditions inside NECC, and had grown angrier with every revelation: the techs wrestling and dry-humping each other; the celebrity names like Miles Davis and RuPaul they'd written on prescriptions in defiance of state inspectors.

Emma Todd died in March 2013 of fungal meningitis after receiving a shot at Michigan Pain Specialists. She'd undergone spinal surgery in an attempt to scrape out the fungus, which had invaded her blood vessels and spinal cord tissue. Her son, Ken, told Strachan that his mother and father had been married for more than sixty years. He'd just finished remodeling his home to make it easier to navigate for his aged parents, who were moving in. Now only his dad was living in the spare room. Recently his dad had looked up at the ceiling with his arms stretched out, and said, "Your mom's here."

Traveling around the country interviewing victims changed how the two prosecutors viewed the case. Strachan knew that thousands of people's lives had been ruined, but listening to Ken Todd's story felt like a giant wave crashing over her. She had to excuse herself to regain a semblance of professional composure.

The prosecutors had met often to debate the charges they would file. Their initial strategy was to charge Cadden with fraud for lying about the quality of his company's drugs. But this case was so big, with so many victims, that fraud could not encompass it.

Earlier in the investigation, the health care group's chief, Nat Yeager, had mentioned to Varghese that he was considering RICO murder charges—the same strategy the office's mob prosecutor had mentioned to Strachan just months into the probe. Strachan had been skeptical; RICO does not cover mere manslaughter or negligence and it would be difficult to prove murderous intent. Varghese, a terrorism and national security prosecutor, saw the path more clearly. He had promised to bring Strachan in on everything. "Nat doesn't want to tell you this, but he's proposed second-degree murder. I think it makes sense," he said. In the corner of his office sat Varghese's whiteboard with lists of illegal practices at NECC, and Strachan stared at it as they talked.

She nodded. "Let's just try our hearts out and see if we get this," she said.

RICO, the Racketeer Influenced and Corrupt Organizations Act, was created in 1970 to allow federal prosecutors to charge the leaders of a criminal enterprise for ordering or aiding in a murder; the capo was still on the hook even if their underlings performed the hit. RICO had been used to charge the Hells Angels, the Gambino crime family, and even a Florida police department that was part of a cocaine ring. But *pharmacists*?

To ask a jury to find a pharmacist guilty of a RICO murder, the evidence had to show that NECC was a criminal enterprise, a racket, and that Cadden and Chin had operated recklessly enough to know that their behavior would kill someone.

After her interviews with the families, any reluctance Strachan had about murder charges had vanished. She believed wholeheartedly that fraud charges alone were not appropriate. In a fraud case, NECC's customers—the clinics, hospitals, and doctors—would be the victims. The jury would never hear the voices of the patients and their loved ones.

In Michigan and six of the other states where people died of fungal meningitis, the second-degree murder statutes outlined a "recklessness" toward human life.

Varghese and Strachan had a direction and strategy. It was time to write the story of their investigation in the form of an indictment. If the grand jury approved it, federal agents could arrest Cadden and the others. But first, they had to present the entire case to the nation's top justice official, Attorney General Eric Holder, for a final approval.

As they wrote what would become a 115-page indictment, they received an emergency alert. Glenn Chin was going to fly to Hong Kong.

SEPTEMBER 2014

LOGAN INTERNATIONAL AIRPORT, BOSTON

The plainclothes agents were indistinguishable from the travelers pulling their luggage through the glass-walled hallways of Logan's international terminal. They waited for the target to clear security so they could move in. Since neither Cadden nor Chin was in custody, the FBI had filed an alert with the Transportation Security Administration for both men. If they did try to fly out of the country, Varghese and Strachan would be alerted.

Just weeks before Varghese and Strachan were scheduled to present their case in Washington, Chin purchased a round-trip ticket from Boston to Hong Kong—a country with veto power over extradition requests by the U.S. He had also booked tickets for his wife, children, and mother-in-law.

Three days before Chin's flight, the prosecutors had to make a decision. Losing one of their two top targets would be devastating. Varghese wanted to keep quiet until the FBI could show up at Logan and arrest him. Strachan thought they should consider talking to Chin's attorney first. But that had risks, too: if he was indeed planning to flee, a heads-up would enable him to evade the federal agents. The FBI reported that both Chin and his wife had family in Hong Kong. The prosecutors drafted a criminal complaint for one count of mail fraud related to the shipment of the methylpred to Michigan, and a judge quickly signed it. They had an arrest warrant.

Chin entered the terminal with his family in tow, dressed like a man going on vacation. The agents waited for him to clear security. They had been instructed to make the arrest discreetly. When Chin's wife and children went to the restroom, they moved in. "We have an arrest warrant for you. Can you please come with us?" Chin came quietly. His family flew to Hong Kong without him.

The agents brought Chin to the federal courthouse, where he was released to home confinement on $50,000 bond. His defense attorney, Paul Shaw, called the arrest "absolute nonsense." Chin was simply going on a family trip to a wedding, he claimed, calling it nothing short of a "publicity stunt" by the government.

NOVEMBER 2014

CONFERENCE ROOM OF THE U.S. ATTORNEY GENERAL

Varghese and Strachan arrived at the Department of Justice's Art Deco headquarters, where they had been scheduled to present the NECC case to Attorney General Holder at ten A.M. But President Obama's defense secretary, Chuck Hagel, was resigning suddenly, and Holder was called away. The presentation would have to wait.

While pacing the hallways, the prosecutors had time to reflect on the previous two years. Strachan, who'd started the case as what she termed the "discovery girl," was about to present the facts of a complex investigation to the attorney general of the United States. Varghese thought there would never be another case more important to him, and was anxious to get to the presentation. NECC was theirs. They were proud of the work they'd done, and eager to share it.

Varghese was also a little annoyed. He thought a visual presentation would be dramatic and impactful, but the nearly century-old conference room that once served as Attorney General Robert Kennedy's office had no screens. So Varghese printed out dozens of copies of the thirty-nine-page presentation. They would have to do it analogue.

Strachan reached into her purse for a piece of gum and felt hard plastic—a Captain America action figure. A good-luck charm. She pulled it out and showed it to Varghese.

Finally, the attorney general was ready. Half a dozen attorneys and their staffs filed in, filling the blue leather chairs around the conference table and along its walls. A short time later, AG Holder and the deputy attorney general, Jim Cole, entered through another door. Holder sat facing Varghese and Strachan.

The room filled with the sound of pages rustling as everyone riffled through their packets, titled "Criminal Investigation of New England Compounding Center." After a few introductions, Strachan began. "We think in order to fully appreciate the gravity of the defendant's criminal conduct, you need to understand the devastation it ultimately caused," she said. "And that starts with the fungal meningitis outbreak, the worst public health crisis caused by a pharmaceutical drug in U.S. history."

The second page displayed three photographs. One was a microscopic image of the scarred spores and wormlike hyphae of *Exserohilum rostratum*. The two others featured petri dishes filled with fuzzy tan and gray growths.

"What you're looking at here are photos of the actual mold found in NECC's preservative-free methylpred," Strachan said. "That grew in people's bodies." The room erupted in groans. "Gross," someone said.

Deputy Attorney General Cole spoke up. "Okay, yes. We'll give you whatever you want. Are we done here?" Everyone laughed, the tense atmosphere dissolved.

Strachan guided them through the case facts: the dozens dead, the hundreds more with fungal infections, meningitis, strokes. The tepid FDA response due to "jurisdictional concerns."

Next Varghese led them through their legal strategy. Over two years, they had executed four search warrants, interviewed 248 witnesses, and issued more than 650 grand jury subpoenas. They'd granted immunity to seven witnesses, including Owen Finnegan, out of the seventy-three who testified. The attorneys flipped to the mug shots of an organizational pyramid of fourteen employees, with Cadden and Chin at the top. "RICO captures the entirety of NECC's criminal activities," Varghese said. It was this criminal enterprise that had unleashed a killer fungus on the nation, and these men had exhibited a depraved indifference to human life.

They would charge twenty-five counts of second-degree in seven states, all tied to people who died after receiving shots, their bodies full of fungus. Any more than that would be too burdensome, they explained, especially on the jury.

When the attorneys flipped the page, a photograph of a bloody brain greeted them. Alice Machowiak had been a widow. She received steroid injections. She died that December, alone. Her niece found her body.

After the meeting, AG Holder told Varghese and Strachan that what they'd just presented was one of the worst criminal acts he'd ever seen. "So I suppose you want me to say yes?" he asked dryly. He approved the case on the spot.

In two weeks, they would present the indictment to the grand jury. They hoped that, finally, Cadden, Chin, and the others would be arrested.

DECEMBER 2014

U.S. ATTORNEY'S OFFICE, BOSTON

Dense fog hung over Boston Harbor and rain pelted the grand jurors as they entered the courthouse. They were there to vote on the indictment. The Department of Justice had planned a press conference with AG Holder, U.S. attorney Carmen Ortiz, and the prosecution team.

Varghese and Strachan were standing in the grand jury room

when the courtroom went dark. The storm had knocked power out
to the entire courthouse. Security was clearing the building; everyone would have to evacuate. They filed into the hallway, a wall of
windows looking out over Boston Harbor, its waters obscured by
the fog.

The prosecutors waited in a courthouse vestibule for two hours,
hoping that the power would come back. Ultimately, the jurors
were sent home. Holder canceled his flight to Boston.

The indictment would have to wait another week.

Cadden knew that his arrest would likely occur on a Wednes-
day. The grand jury met on Tuesdays, which meant that any
indictment would be filed on that day. The arrest would come next.

His lawyer, Bruce Singal, had been a federal prosecutor in the
1980s, working in the Boston U.S. Attorney's Office alongside
Robert Mueller. His last case was a victory, defending the general
manager of a company who faced up to nine years in prison after a
jury found him guilty of providing shoddy concrete to the city
during its "Big Dig," one of the costliest and most corruption-
riddled public works projects in U.S. history. Singal's client, Robert
Prosperi, instead received a sentence of six months of home confinement, 1,000 hours of community service, and two years' probation.

Cadden's legal strategy would be to point the finger at Chin. The
NECC-funded attorney who represented Chin after his airport arrest had left the case after the Conigliaros stopped paying. Chin
received a court-appointed lawyer, Stephen Weymouth, who worked
out of a shabby office near downtown and had never tried a case of
such magnitude.

A week after the power outage, the grand jury reassembled. Finally, after years of investigation and delays, the prosecutors had their indictment. It charged Cadden, Chin, and twelve other NECC employees and owners, including co-owners Dr. Douglas and Carla Conigliaro; the building's owner and NECC executive Greg Conigliaro; sales director Rob Ronzio; pharmacists Gene Svirskiy, Chris Leary, Joseph Evanosky, and the tech working without a license, Scott "Mudgum" Connolly; and Cadden's operations chief, Sharon Carter.

Cadden and Chin were charged with second-degree murder under RICO. The grand jury process is secret, so the defense attorneys had not been privy to the prosecutors' strategy. They'd been ready for a cascade of fraud charges—not murder.

The next day, Cadden woke up at four A.M. in his Wrentham mansion and got dressed in jeans and a button-down shirt. He took his dog for a walk. The previous week's canceled press conference had local reporters on alert. A television station staked out Cadden's house to get shots of the arrest. The cameras captured him standing with his dog, paper coffee cup in hand. Afterward, he waited in his kitchen for the FBI to arrive.

For Chin, the arrest was a surprise. Steve Weymouth had been on the case for only two months and had not informed his client that the feds were coming. He was still dressed for bed, in an old Patriots T-shirt and pajama bottoms. Teams of federal agents simultaneously moved in on the Conigliaros, Sharon Carter, and the pharmacists charged.

Varghese and Strachan sat in the conference room where they'd interviewed Finnegan and other witnesses, monitoring the arrests in real time. Voices crackled over the radio as the teams confirmed that they had their targets in custody.

More than two years after the outbreak began, Cadden was finally under arrest. When the last FBI agent called in, Strachan felt a weight lift. The investigation had been like hitting one brick wall after another, from being stonewalled by public health agencies on victim identifications to Chin's attempted break for Hong Kong.

Outside the federal courthouse, reporters asked Cadden's attorney, Bruce Singal, for a response. He said Cadden was looking forward to his day in court.

CHAPTER 13

TRIAL

JANUARY 2017

JOHN JOSEPH MOAKLEY UNITED STATES COURTHOUSE, BOSTON

Twelve men and women trudged through snow and ice toward the hulking brick and glass building. Chosen from hundreds of citizens, these jurors would decide Cadden's fate. Among them was an office manager at a surgeon's office, a chef, and a local politician. It was a murder case unlike any that had been heard before, even here in one of the oldest district courts in the country, founded in 1789.

The freeze slowed Boston's finicky public rail system, the T, and one juror was late. As Judge Richard Stearns took his seat, he put the tardy juror at ease. "Don't feel bad, every jury in the courthouse is having problems this morning because of the commuter rail," he said. "It was nobody's fault, and we're all together, and we're ready to start."

It had been a little more than four years since Tom Rybinski appeared at Vanderbilt University Medical Center in Nashville with a rare form of meningitis, the beginning of a disease outbreak that became the worst of its kind. The government had filed ninety-seven felony counts against Barry Cadden, including twenty-five second-degree murders and hundreds of criminal charges against thirteen other NECC owners and employees. This was the first in a series of trials that would stretch over the next two years. The stakes were high for Cadden and his attorneys, Bruce Singal and Michelle Peirce. If convicted of murder, Cadden would spend the rest of his life in a federal prison. For Varghese and Strachan, it was the first test of whether the government's decision to use the RICO statute would prove wise.

Varghese's opening statement would be the first time the government described the case in public, and he was tight with nerves. The previous Friday, he had practiced for Strachan, their paralegal, the health care unit chief Nat Yeager, and the six law clerks working with them. His remarks were too long, so he spent the weekend editing, revising, and memorizing. He recited them again for his wife, Carole, who fell asleep ten minutes in. The morning of the trial, he was still murmuring it to himself while walking his dog. Strachan told him he was ready.

Varghese arrived early to set up his slide presentation. But he had to wait for the last juror to arrive. He paced in the hallway and practiced again for a colleague. At last the jury was seated.

The courtroom was standing room only with reporters, FBI investigators, and fungal meningitis patients and their family members. Two overflow rooms with video feeds were also filled to capacity with more media and defense lawyers representing the other NECC clients. Notably absent were Cadden's wife and children. He was alone.

Judge Stearns motioned to the prosecution to begin. This moment was more than four years in the making, during which Varghese had absorbed all the arcane bits of evidence and how they fit together to tell a story. He was wearing the sage-green tie he called his "closing tie" and he was pulsing with adrenaline. He launched the presentation on a laptop and reached for the remote.

The screens filled with a photograph of a bespectacled man with a kind smile standing with his arm around a young woman. "Douglas Wingate, a forty-seven-year-old accountant at Pepsi, a husband, a father of two, walked into a medical clinic in Roanoke, Virginia, known as Insight Imaging. He was going there because in a couple of weeks he was about to leave on a cruise to go to the Bahamas with his wife, Sharon. They were going to celebrate their twenty-fifth wedding anniversary. On that day, September 6, 2012, he got the shot in his back and he went home," Varghese said.

Within days, Wingate was unresponsive. He could not recognize his wife, Varghese explained. "He lingered for a few more days and he died. He died on September 18, 2012, twelve days after receiving that steroid injection in his back." Varghese clicked to the next photograph, of an elderly black man in Florida named Godwin Mitchell, who'd also received a shot for back pain. He was playing the harmonica when he had a stroke, before a painful decline into death.

Varghese pointed to Cadden, sitting next to his attorneys, an electric monitor strapped to his ankle.

"This is Barry Cadden, and he ran a company called NECC," Varghese said. "Barry Cadden was the owner. He was the president. He was the head pharmacist. Barry Cadden was NECC."

The screens displayed a brain and spinal cord floating in black space. A syringe zoomed into view, the animation showing an injection. Black specks representing mold spores appeared in the spine, and the injection site turned crimson to represent the fungus's spread upward, the spine looking like an overheated thermometer as the infection climbed toward the brain. "When it was deposited in the epidural space, that fungus ate through and entered into what's known as the cerebrospinal fluid," Varghese said. "This fungus is what's called angiophilic. That means it likes to eat blood vessels. When the fungus reaches the base of your brain, it ate through the blood vessels and caused a massive stroke."

He again motioned toward the defense table. "They were making drugs, and it's high-risk because they were taking non-sterile ingredients to make a sterile drug. This was NECC's business. Their job was to make sure that these drugs were sterile. That's what it means to be a high-risk compounder."

A photograph of one of NECC's vials of milky methylprednisolone appeared. Near the top of the vial, where the glass curved into the jar's capstem, a black smudge clung to the inside. "That's the mold that was in the drugs that killed," Varghese said.

The next slide showed an overhead photo of a petri dish with furry circles of mold. "That was the mold placed in the epidural space, and that was the mold that made its way to their brains and ultimately caused their deaths," Varghese said, his voice rising. The courtroom was silent.

"NECC and Barry Cadden sent out 17,600 vials contaminated with this mold. 17,600 vials to twenty-three different states," he continued. "It was the largest public health crisis ever [caused] by a pharmaceutical drug."

Then the picture of a fax. "This is an actual order form that came into NECC. Look at the names: L.L. Bean, Filet O'fish. That's not even a person. That's a sandwich," Varghese said, laughs from the jury box cutting through the tension. "Harry Potter, Coco Puff. Drugs kept shipping."

"They were counting on the fact that the regulators wouldn't look close enough to find Filet O'fish and L.L. Bean," Varghese said.

For the jurors to believe Cadden committed murder, they would first have to find him guilty of RICO violations, or running an illegal racket. Varghese focused much of his opening statement on the elements of NECC's operations that showed an institutional recklessness. If the jury agreed that NECC had operated as a criminal organization, then they might believe that Cadden exhibited a "depraved indifference" for human life, the definition of second-degree murder in most states.

Proving this beyond a reasonable doubt would not be easy. Cadden did not work in the clean room. He had not mixed the drugs. But Varghese and Strachan believed that focusing on Cadden's greed would show jurors that he prized profit over patient safety—evidence of the willful, reckless disregard for the people receiving his company's medications. They would also present evidence that Cadden withheld vital information about the quickly escalating catastrophe from the CDC, endangering more lives.

Varghese launched into more stories of the victims. "You're going to hear over the next few weeks about twenty-five people who died because of these drugs. Let me introduce you to them." A smiling blond woman's photo filled the screen. "Kathy Sinclair was from Roanoke, Virginia," he said. "Tom Rybinski from Tennessee. Judge Eddie Lovelace. He was from Kentucky." He ended with Lyn Laperriere in Michigan.

"You're going to hear that there is no natural way for fungus to actually get into your brain, unless it gets put there," Varghese said. "Unless . . . it's put there, and it gets into the cerebrospinal fluid and makes its way there like in this case."

During the early days, doctors asked Cadden directly if patients were being harmed by his products. "He said no. At that point he knew people were getting sick. At that point he knew people might die. He said no," Varghese said somberly. "Every single minute mattered, every single day mattered, and Barry Cadden could only think of himself and his baby, NECC."

Bruce Singal stood at the lectern, facing the jury. "Let me tell you, there is no monopoly in this courtroom on the compassion and the empathy for these poor people and what they have suffered through," he began. "It's not exclusively in the government's possession."

Cadden's defense team believed that the government's road to a murder conviction rested in large part with the emotional testimony of the victims' families. During pretrial hearings they asked Judge Stearns to toss out the murder charges; without them, the family members could not testify. Even though he voiced skepticism of the government's indictment, Judge Stearns allowed the murder charges to proceed. The jury would be the final arbiter.

Plan B was to limit victims' testimony as much as possible. To do this, Cadden's team did not contest the fact that NECC's drugs had caused their loved ones' deaths. This removed the need for lengthy medical examiner testimony about the excruciating ways in which they had died. One examiner could testify toward all twenty-five alleged murders. It also limited the number of family members from whom the jury would hear.

Singal attacked the prosecutors as overzealous. A veteran lawyer with decades in the federal courts, he said the ambitious prosecutors had been too influenced by the victims' stories and had overcharged the case. "Barry Cadden is charged with murdering these people. . . . The very worst thing you can accuse somebody of, ladies and gentlemen, is murder, and they have accused him of it twenty-five times," he said with a tone of incredulity.

It is the job of prosecutors to prove facts, and of the defense to create doubt about those facts. "We don't have to prove anything," Singal added. "But we will prove a bunch of things in this case, and . . . one of the things we're going to prove is that Barry Cadden did not murder these twenty-five individuals."

The defense needed someone to shoulder the blame. Chin topped their list of targets. He made the drugs and faced the same murder charges as Cadden. His trial was the next one scheduled, and it was clear from his pretrial filings that Chin's team would return the favor and point to Cadden as the architect.

Singal brought out an organizational chart of NECC. Cadden's photo was at the top of the pyramid. "In addition to Mr. Chin as the head of the whole clean operation . . . you had all the pharmacy techs who were under them, and then in addition to that you had pharmacists who were inspecting the drug before it went out." The prosecutors were "misstating the evidence and giving you a distorted picture of Barry Cadden and of NECC." Strachan's expression tightened.

Singal then played a recording of a voice mail, the audio cutting through the quiet courtroom. "Hello, this is Barry Cadden from New England Compounding Center, your facility's source of medication from us for methylprednisolone acetate. . . . We received a complaint from a client late this past evening of potential foreign particulates in a number of vials they received. We would like you to quarantine this product at this point. Call us as soon as possible to discuss the situation. We consider this an emergency, so please, if you get this message, transfer to the individual in charge of medications."

Singal sought to raise doubt that Cadden acted with a depraved heart. "Listen to [Cadden's] actual words on this tape recording because that reflects the heart and mind of that individual, not the words you heard from Mr. Varghese," Singal said.

D r. Ben Park was nervous. He'd never testified in a criminal trial before, let alone a murder case. He worried about the cross-examination from Cadden's defense attorneys—how in movies they always skewer the witnesses, tripping them up with tricky questions and making them look foolish. One of the attorneys gave him a piece of advice: Don't let the defense trap you. Just say what you want to say. Take control of the message.

Park was the government's first witness, there to testify about the breadth and scope of the outbreak. The judge had limited Varghese and Strachan's discussion of the epidemic—it would come directly from the experts and a few victim witnesses. Park would be the first to tell the jury what had happened. He waited in a vestibule off the courtroom while the attorneys delivered their openings. He tried meditating and deep breathing to get his thoughts in order. When he was called in, he walked down the center aisle to the witness stand.

Park's voice quivered as he introduced himself. Varghese asked him to slow down. "Okay. I'm excited. Sorry," Park said.

He began again. He spoke directly to Varghese, telling him how the early cases in Tennessee had mystified the CDC. He described the moment when he learned that the disease was infecting people in other states, and how he scrambled to find the source. While the agency always suspected NECC's steroids, it required weeks of investigation to confirm.

Park glanced at Cadden and said that he reached out to learn about any contamination concerns at NECC.

"They said they had not had any issues with any environmental concerns."

"Why were you asking that question?"

"We wanted to know if they had had any indication that there could be a contamination."

"Would that have made a difference in terms of your investigation?"

"It would have raised our suspicion that the product was the culprit."

"So, Dr. Park, in your experience, can you tell us how significant was this outbreak?"

Park gave the CDC's overview of the outbreak: the dozens of dead and the hundreds infected. The attorneys on both sides noticed that jurors were paying rapt attention, crinkling their faces in disgust or furrowing their brows with seeming disbelief as he spoke.

"In my fifteen years being at CDC investigating outbreaks, the only thing that rises to this level was the Ebola epidemic," he said. "But this one was here in our country and was entirely preventable."

Bruce Singal describes a trial as "armed combat," and lawyers as "soldiers and scholars" on the courtroom battlefield. One weapon for a defense attorney is to disrupt the prosecution's rhythm. Varghese started with an emotional opening statement and an impressive witness; Singal wanted to slow things down. He and Peirce interrupted with constant objections, followed by meandering cross-examinations that drew Judge Stearns's censure and looks of tired resignation from the jury.

The trial slowed to a mind-numbing pace. As Peirce cross-examined Park about the minutiae of how the CDC tested for mold in the samples collected from fungal meningitis patients, she cut him off mid-sentence, peppering him with leading questions.

"So the concern in that email is [that] it's possible that the testing process itself is producing certain mold or other organism that get sent to CDC?"

"Routinely, what we do . . ."

"Is that the concern that you're expressing in that email, to be sure that we understand whether the labs themselves are contaminating the samples?"

"This is routine. We always confirm findings so . . ."

"You always do that because it's always possible that lab personnel themselves might themselves put a fungus in the sample when they're testing, not intentionally, of course."

"I'm sorry, the question is why do we confirm this?"

Park was the first of fifty-nine prosecution witnesses. It would take almost two full days to get through his testimony.

TRIAL DAY 10

Collette Rybinski's voice was shaky as she took the oath. Because her husband, Tom, was the index case, interview requests had poured in after news of Cadden's arrest broke. Camera crews camped outside her house. Still consumed by grief, she tired quickly of the attention and had been reluctant to talk with the prosecution. Strachan convinced her to participate in the case.

Varghese and Strachan had agreed that they wanted jurors to hear from each of them equally during the trial. They chose their interviews based on their rapport with particular witnesses—Varghese with Owen Finnegan, Strachan with the wives who had lost their husbands.

Questioning a victim's family member in a murder trial is always a tightrope walk. Collette was the first of three victims' relatives Strachan would be allowed to call to the stand, and she wanted to set the right tone. These stories showed the real toll of NECC's hubris and greed, but they could seem exploitative and risked angering the judge and jury. Strachan resolved to keep the testimony brief while still bringing Tom Rybinski to life so the jurors would feel the same emotional impact she'd experienced during her victim interviews.

As a photograph of Tom flashed on the display, Collette described how they had met a few years earlier at a songwriters' music club outside Nashville. Tom was adventurous and quick-witted, only slowed a bit by a herniated disk in his lower back, for which he'd received the methylprednisolone acetate shots. The steroids relieved his pain, so Collette and he rarely discussed it. Then she described the horror of his deterioration as the meningitis took hold. The last moment that Tom communicated with her, they had been watching a show about Alaska in his hospital room. The courtroom fell silent.

"I said, 'Do you remember Alaska? Do you remember going to Alaska?'" Collette said. "He shook his head no. And I said, 'You don't remember going—being there?' And he said, 'No.' And I said, 'That was our honeymoon. You don't remember the honeymoon?' . . . And I said, 'Well, if you don't—do you remember getting married?' He shook his head no. And I said, 'Well, if you don't remember our honeymoon and you don't remember getting married, why do you always know when the doctors ask who I am? How do you always know I'm your wife?' And he turned around and he looked at me and he said, 'Because I know.'"

By the end of her thirty-minute testimony, several jurors were in tears.

The judge looked over at the defense table.

"No questions, Your Honor," Singal said.

TRIAL DAY 14

In the third week of testimony, the jury was getting visibly and audibly cranky. The previous witness, NECC pharmacy technician Joe Connolly, had testified about the shortcuts and the testosterone-fueled culture that dominated the clean room. Peirce objected to almost every one of the prosecution's questions, which sometimes required Judge Stearns to halt the testimony to advise the jury about points of law. During her cross-examination, Peirce spent nearly two full days asking the same questions, diving into details of a drug's recipe worksheet over and over again.

The judge called the attorneys aside with a warning. The jurors were complaining. "They are being driven crazy by the repetition. They said, 'Look, we're taking notes. We're intelligent people. Why are they treating us like children?'"

He turned to Varghese and Strachan. "I think you better think on the government's side about compressing this case because, as they said, 'Is their strategy to bore us to death?' Those were their exact words. So, just by way of caution."

O wen Finnegan was at a urinal when he heard a voice: "Hey, OJ, what's going on?" It was Cadden. He went to the stall next to Finnegan. "How's it going?" Finnegan couldn't believe Cadden was making small talk, just before he was to testify at Cadden's murder trial. "What are you doing now?" Cadden asked. Finnegan told him he'd gotten a job at a used-car dealership. Cadden was familiar with the place. "You know a guy, Clemmy, over there?" he asked. Finnegan nodded. "Oh yeah, he and I been friends a long time," Cadden said. After a few minutes of small talk, Cadden left. Finnegan chuckled to himself. *Surreal,* he thought. Cadden hadn't changed a bit.

On the witness stand, as Finnegan grasped the jug of water to fill his glass, he saw that his hand was shaking. Under questioning by Varghese, he described a clean-room culture that was anything but clean: the horseplay, the cut corners, the walking around without booties. From time to time, Finnegan looked at Cadden but his old boss mostly stared at the table in front of him.

Varghese pulled up various tests that identified mold and bacterial growths throughout 2012, some on Finnegan's workstation. "To your knowledge, was anything done when environmental monitoring hits came back?" Varghese asked. While the pace had picked up slightly after Judge Stearns's warning, Singal objected. Stearns allowed Finnegan to answer.

"There were times when Glenn would tell you, 'Hey, look, you popped off'—popped off, meaning you had either bacteria or something else came up back on the petri dish," Finnegan responded.

"Was anything recleaned?"

"No."

TRIAL DAY 24

In Boston, one entity eclipses all others, even a federal murder trial. The twenty-fourth day of testimony was disrupted by a victory parade for the New England Patriots, who had just won the Super Bowl. Public transit was a mess. With more than a month to go, Judge Stearns was still worried about the jury's attention span. "There must be thousands of people employed making 'Brady' jerseys, from what I saw this morning. It's going to be hard for him to find his real one," he quipped.

Varghese and Strachan had a significant setback the day before, when Judge Stearns sided with the defense and forbade the prosecutors from calling any more family members to the stand. Testimony from Collette Rybinski, Sharon Wingate, and the son of a third victim from Maryland, Bahman Kashi, had clearly moved the jury, and the defense argued it was prejudicial. Judge Stearns was skeptical that more testimony from victims would give the jurors information they did not already have.

Stearns had already excluded autopsy photos, except for microscopic images of *E. rostratum* in the body, and now the victims' nightmarish stories would be limited. With weeks left to go, by the end of the trial, the impact of the testimony from those who had been affected would have faded.

TRIAL DAY 28

Strachan and Varghese still needed to address their most pressing question: How did the mold get into NECC's drugs? The extent of the contamination at NECC was clear, but neither the CDC nor the FDA could say for certain how *Exserohilum rostratum* had ended up inside the individual vials. It was a blind spot that Cadden's defense exploited to raise doubt. Annette Robinson, disheveled and anxious as she was, would be the prosecutors' best shot at clarifying that the building and clean room where NECC made its drugs was regularly contaminated with mold.

Strachan displayed a document for the jury, "Standard Operating Procedure for Quality Check and Vetting of Patient Names." It laid out the ways in which NECC was supposed to ensure they were making drugs based on real prescriptions. Robinson's job had been to police these rules. Strachan asked about the document. "I've never seen this before," Robinson said. "I don't even know what vetting means."

Cadden had hired Robinson to help ensure that NECC's clean rooms were sterile and that its pharmacists followed the law. The fact that she was entirely unqualified, and that her oversight included allowing the pharmacists to accept clearly fake names, was a convincing indication of Cadden's recklessness. Strachan asked Robinson if she could remember any of the made-up names.

"Anita Knapp." Robinson giggled. She especially liked that one, "because I like to take naps so . . . And then [there] was like Mickey Mouse and Donald Duck and Michael Jackson. Those kinds of names."

On July 5 and again a week later, July 12, Robinson had found "overgrown mold" on a sample taken from the shelves where Chin stored methylpred and the container that Finnegan used to fill the vials. This was the closest the prosecution had gotten to tying the mold found in the clean room to the drugs that had killed so many people. In fact, Robinson red-flagged mold hits almost weekly. But production never stopped.

The defense team moved in, seeking to damage Robinson's already shaky credibility. Peirce highlighted her errors on the stand: she'd confused the term *humidity* with temperature, for one. Then Peirce questioned her testing results. Robinson grew defiant as the questioning got heated.

"So you would get samples from a particular lot, correct? I just want to make sure people know what a stability study is," Peirce asked.

"I don't really know what you're saying. From a specific lot?"

"So—"

"I'm not understanding you," Robinson interrupted.

"When you said you would ship them out, am I correct that what you would do is send samples from the same lot over time, so thirty days, sixty days, and the potency would be tested?"

"You didn't say that before."

"I'm trying to clarify what I said."

"That's a yes," Robinson said.

Robinson had testified for three days, during which Judge Stearns warned Peirce about her aggression toward the witness. "All right. Jurors, perhaps mercifully, it's 1:00. Don't forget it's a three-day weekend," he said, and adjourned.

TRIAL DAY 38

Rob Ronzio entered the courtroom looking fit, his dark hair gelled firmly in place. The jury had heard from Finnegan and others who worked with Chin in the clean room, but none was as close to Cadden as Ronzio. The sales director's testimony would be key to substantiating the murder charges and the prosecution's theory that Cadden was more concerned about damage control than warning patients.

Ronzio's cooperation was an eleventh-hour coup for the prosecutors. Since the indictment, he had refused to speak with the government on the advice of an attorney he'd been given through NECC. But two weeks before the trial, and with a new attorney, he pleaded guilty and entered into an agreement to testify against his former colleagues.

Ronzio settled into his seat on the witness stand. Varghese described the plea and cooperation agreements. He wanted to confront any potential questions about Ronzio's credibility up front, telling the jury that no promises had been made in connection with his testimony.

The defense cried foul immediately, seeking to cast Ronzio as self-serving and unreliable. They complained that they had received a memo from the government only days before the trial started with the details of Ronzio's statement. They wanted the government's notes from its preparation interviews, too.

Judge Stearns's patience was wearing thin. "I mean, you're a trial lawyer," he said to Singal. "You're surprised by a witness? What is the surprise in that? That's what trials are about." Motion denied.

Ronzio spoke assuredly. He sent salesman Mario Giamei to Nashville to meet with the staff at the St. Thomas Outpatient Neurosurgical Center when the first meningitis cases surfaced. Cadden had fumed, complaining that the visit could muddy a delicate legal matter.

"Did you have any conversations with Mr. Cadden on Monday, September 24, about the complaint and what seemed to be the issue?" Varghese asked.

"When it first happened, he said: 'It's us.' He knew right away it was us."

"What was your response when he said: 'It's us'?"

"I still couldn't believe it was us, and I said, 'Well, Barry, let's look at all the other potential scenarios during the procedure.'"

Cadden's reluctance to warn others about what he himself suspected spoke to his depraved indifference, the prosecutors believed. For dozens of patients who were starting to feel dizziness and other meningitis symptoms as Cadden weighed his options, every passing hour affected life-and-death decisions by their doctors.

Varghese asked Ronzio to read an email from the concerned nurse in Indiana, which he had received the evening after the CDC call and Cadden's email to Ronzio in response: "Oh, no."

It was strong evidence, made available only because Ronzio had agreed to testify. In cross-examination, Peirce told the jury that Ronzio had likely escaped a five-year federal prison sentence with this deal.

"The timing is important because you're of more use to the government, aren't you, prior to Mr. Cadden's trial than if you approached them to plead guilty after; isn't that right?" she asked.

"I believe that's a question for the government," Ronzio replied.

"Well, it's a question for you, Mr. Ronzio."

Peirce questioned Ronzio's memory of the dates when he'd heard Cadden say "it's us," insinuating that he'd only remembered an earlier date because it was what the government wanted to hear.

"I wanted to take responsibility," Ronzio responded. "And I wanted the opportunity to speak."

TRIAL DAY 46

Strachan was wearing a white tweed blazer over a black dress, clothes she'd purchased just for this moment. The colors communicated good and evil, she thought. She took a breath and reminded herself of everything that had happened to land her here in front of the jury. Five years earlier, she had been handling discovery for the government's legal team. Now she was its closer. She had spent months practicing, running through her arguments during yoga class, tapping out notes on her phone while jogging, testing out her ideas on Uber drivers.

After forty-five days of grinding, hard-fought testimony, each side was entitled to give a closing argument to frame the evidence their way. Closing arguments are, by design, more difficult for the prosecution. The defense just needs to convince one juror to see things their way, while prosecutors need unanimity to convict.

The courtroom fell silent. "We made it," she said with a grin, looking at the jury. "Unlike when we started this journey, this time I have a voice. And it will probably not surprise you to hear that this is a good thing because I have some things to say.

"Let me ask you this: Have you ever stopped to think about all of the things that NECC did wrong?" Strachan practically vibrated with urgency as she ticked off the elements of the prosecution's key argument: NECC was a racket, and a murderous one.

"They shipped the drug without prescriptions. They shipped drugs with expired ingredients. They ignored environmental monitoring results showing mold and bacteria in that clean room. Cadden made misrepresentations to the regulators. He made misrepresentations to the customers. He made misrepresentations to the sales reps that he trained."

The jury was paying attention, Strachan thought. She pivoted to the government's marquee criminal charges. The jury had to understand why this was reckless murder, not just negligent sloppiness.

"He knew the injectable drugs that he was making would kill people if they were contaminated, but he kept making them anyway without taking the necessary steps to ensure that they were sterile," she said, motioning toward the expressionless Cadden.

She paused.

"That is a wanton and willful disregard for patients' lives. That is a depraved indifference for human life, for the lives of twenty-five people who trusted that the drugs he was making were safe."

Strachan displayed photos of the NECC salesmen who had testified. She reminded the jury of how Cadden had trained them to peddle their drugs to hospitals and doctors, maintaining that the company exceeded the U.S. Pharmacopeia's sterility standards when he knew it did not. He was selling the company as the "Ferrari of Compounders" when it was just a small group of overworked pharmacists and techs in a warehouse next to a recycling plant holding old mattresses and other trash—a breeding ground for mold and bacteria.

She clicked over to mug shots of Finnegan and the other technicians. "They told you about all of the different ways that NECC's clean-room operations fell far short of what regulations required. While the sales reps had no idea what was going on in the lab, after nine weeks, you do."

The contaminated batches that spawned the fungal meningitis outbreak were mixtures of old and new stock chemicals—the "botching lots." "Members of the jury, this matters," she said. "When the outbreak hit and CDC was rapidly responding, they needed to know who received which lots, and mixed lots can't be traced. If the lot number is meaningless, how do you know what you sent and what was used?"

The screen filled with a calendar that was a patchwork of color. Each month displayed at least one red day when Robinson's monitoring found mold—seventy in all. "Here's the real picture about what NECC looked like in 2012," Strachan said, gesturing toward the image, the red days giving jurors the impression of a company under siege. It also showed the dates that the drugs were shipped.

Strachan paused as she brought up text from the U.S. Pharmacopeia. "That danger is even greater when fungi are involved. That *Exserohilum rostratum* that was growing in the room in June and got into the lot was still growing in the room in August, two months later. And then it grew in patients' bodies," she said.

A photograph of the CDC's Dr. Ben Park. "He told you it was critical to get the word out so that patients could look for symptoms and he could save lives, because they identified quickly in the beginning that 50 percent of the patients were dying.

"Barry Cadden knew what would happen at NECC if he didn't do things right. He knew, but he still ran NECC the way he did. He never stopped drug production for a day."

Finally, she showed photos of the twenty-five victims for which Cadden faced murder charges. Strachan read their names and asked for convictions on all counts. Her closing lasted ninety minutes.

When the jury returned from break, Bruce Singal was waiting for them.

"This is indeed a tragic death case, but it is not a murder case. And there is a big, big difference between the two."

The government was overreaching, he argued. "That mystery as to how the contamination was caused, ladies and gentlemen, regrettably remains unsolved as we sit here today. And without having solved it, there is no way that Mr. Cadden can be convicted of second-degree murder, I would suggest, especially in the absence of any evidence otherwise linking him to the deaths of these people.

"What we have seen, ladies and gentlemen, is a prosecution by deception and by distortion," Singal said. "If you go around the corner in this building, you'll see there are signs. If you take a right out the front door, there's a quotation from [former U.S. Supreme Court Associate Justice Felix] Frankfurter. It reads, 'The responsibility of those who exercise power in a democratic government is not to reflect inflamed public feeling but to help form its understanding.' And I would suggest to you, ladies and gentlemen, that this case has undermined that rule and is inflaming public feeling without contributing to understanding, in effect, distorting understanding."

Strachan shook her head slightly as Varghese rose to deliver a rebuttal.

"Let me just go over a couple of things that Mr. Singal said, because the truth is, what he just did was stand up before you and make excuses and misleading statements about the evidence in this case. And you know that because you know the truth.

"Why were those drugs contaminated? Because they started out that way. His job was to make sure that those drugs were sterile before anybody got injected with them," Varghese said, pointing at Cadden.

"You know that in 2012, when production ramped up, when cleaning dropped, and when mold was prevalent throughout the clean room, it was no longer a simple game of Russian roulette. The odds increased. He was putting more bullets in the gun."

Varghese returned to his seat.

"I'm afraid the drama is over," Judge Stearns said. After lunch, the jury would receive their instructions. One point was the very foundation of the American justice system: "A defendant is innocent in the eyes of the law unless and until you, as the jury, decide unanimously that the government has proved his guilt beyond a reasonable doubt."

Varghese and Strachan had worked for nearly five years on the case. Now it was out of their hands.

* * *

In the deliberation room, juror Melanie Gomes stood up, a dictionary in her hand. She'd been going over the definitions of *reckless* and *wanton*, words used to describe second-degree murder in states where the victims had died. She was troubled by those words and did not think the government had proved that Cadden himself was reckless or had acted with a wanton disregard for human life. They'd shown that Cadden was a negligent businessman, sure—but a murderer?

Gomes was in the minority. Most of the jurors, including the foreman, Richard Hill, favored finding Cadden guilty on the majority of the twenty-five murder charges. A few others were not sure. Gomes wanted to be dispassionate, and the prosecution's attempts to sway her emotions had not landed. Something was missing.

The jury had been tight knit since the start of the trial. They had nicknames for the lawyers. Singal was Mr. Rogers. Strachan the Bulldog. But now they were arguing, crying. People kept changing their minds.

Hill kept a running tab on the splits. A majority favored guilty verdicts on twenty-one murders. Some counts were nine to three, or eight to four, or seven to five. Everyone agreed, because of the wording, that Florida's and North Carolina's murder statutes did not apply to Cadden, so they had a unanimous vote to acquit on those two counts. They voted nine to three to acquit on Virginia's, too.

Gomes remained firmly in the not-guilty group for murder across the board. She argued that the consequences of the outbreak were a result of a systemic collapse, not one person's fault. Regulators who turned a blind eye. Doctors who benefited from buying cheaper drugs. The private drug-testing lab—Analytical Research Laboratories in Oklahoma—that NECC sometimes used, which also did not detect a fungal contaminant until it was too late. Cadden was guilty of manslaughter from negligence, but that was not an option.

To convict on murder they had to agree unanimously that Cadden knew that operating NECC so recklessly would result in patient deaths. At least nine jurors were certain that he did and were ready to move forward. But Gomes, and two of her peers, refused to budge.

MARCH 2017

COURTROOM NO. 21, U.S. DISTRICT COURT, BOSTON

Strachan's phone rang. It was Judge Stearns's clerk. After three days of deliberations, the jury had reached a verdict. They had twenty minutes to get to the courthouse.

Word quickly spread to the press and the small community of attorneys in Boston, many of whom began to stream through the courthouse metal detectors.

A cold wind hit Varghese and Strachan as they walked over the Seaport Boulevard bridge and turned left on Sleeper Street. Strachan's heart was in her throat. "Is this going to be okay?" she asked.

"It's definitely not going to be an acquittal," Varghese said. He'd seen a few jurors visibly moved by Strachan's closing argument, and he was confident that they had Cadden on mail fraud at the very least. "They might hang," he said. A hung jury would give them a chance to make adjustments and try again. "But definitely not an acquittal."

"All rise," the clerk bellowed as Judge Stearns entered from his chambers. The judge explained that the verdict slip would be handed to him first. "It will take me several minutes to verify that the slip is filled out properly."

"All rise for the jury," the clerk intoned. The onlookers in the seating gallery shot up, the rumble and creak of the wooden benches filling the room.

The jury filed in. Judge Stearns asked if they had reached a verdict. "That's correct," Hill said, handing over the verdict slip. The room was silent save for the rustle of pages as the judge read through the ninety-seven counts. Varghese kept his eyes glued to a copy of the verdict slip on the tabletop in front of him.

Finally Judge Stearns looked up. "The verdict slip is in order. It has been very carefully filled out," he said. He handed it back to the clerk.

The clerk looked at the judge. "What about these numbers?" she asked.

Varghese turned to Strachan and mouthed "Numbers? Why are there numbers?" In his twelve years as a federal prosecutor he'd never seen a verdict form with numbers. The jury foreperson is only supposed to check "guilty" or "not guilty." Numbers indicated a lack of unanimity—a split.

"In some cases on the verdict slip—it will become part of the public record—the jurors indicate how they voted in terms of a division. That need not be read, just the verdict itself," the judge said.

Before Varghese and Strachan could parse the meaning of the split, the clerk began reading. The first twenty-seven charges were for racketeering. They needed guilty verdicts to get the murders. It could all be over before it started.

"Racketeering Act 1: Guilty."

Varghese exhaled.

Guilty. Guilty. Guilty. Twenty-six more times, guilty of racketeering and mail fraud. Cadden showed no emotion as the clerk moved on.

Racketeering Act 28, Murder of Karina Baxter. "Not guilty," the clerk said.

Strachan hung her head and shook it, trying to keep her composure.

Count 29, the murder of Paula Brent. Not guilty.

Racketeering Act Number 37, Murder of Eddie Lovelace. Not guilty.

Racketeering Act Number 40, Murder of Thomas Rybinski. Not guilty.

Barry Cadden was guilty of charges related to running a criminal business, shipping untested drugs, using an unlicensed pharmacy technician to make medicines, introducing misbranded drugs into interstate commerce with intent to defraud and mislead, and mail fraud. But he was not guilty of the twenty-five murders, or for shipping expired drugs.

The verdict was a mixed bag, with victories for both sides. But there was no doubt that Cadden had won the most pivotal contest of the day. His team left the courthouse triumphantly. They'd spared their client a life sentence. Even though he still faced a maximum sentence of more than thirty years, they'd done their job. The verdict confirmed their argument that the government had overcharged.

A throng had gathered outside. "Murder is the worst crime known to humanity, and it is a crime that Barry Cadden was labeled with this charge for more than two years," Singal told a reporter for Boston public radio station WBUR. "It is a disgrace that he was charged with murder. It is unprovable, unwarranted, and unjustified. And we are deeply grateful that the jury saw it that way and vindicated Mr. Cadden on all twenty-five of the murder charges."

Inside, Varghese and Strachan seethed. They asked the clerk for a copy of the verdict slip and staked an attorney outside the courtroom door to wait for it. They had to see the numbers for themselves. They'd gotten Cadden on dozens of charges, but it felt like the judge had stolen their victory by not ordering the jury to continue deliberating after seeing the vote counts. When the form finally arrived, it confirmed their suspicions: a majority of the jurors had wanted to vote guilty on twenty-one of the murder counts.

Strachan was exhausted. On her office door, her clerks had taped a life-sized poster of Patriots head coach Bill Belichick. The coach was standing outside after a game, his dark hair matted to his head from a steady rain. He looked determined. In bold white letters it read *We're on to Cincinnati*.

The Cincinnati quote was a myth-making one. In 2014, the Patriots had just been slaughtered by the Kansas City Chiefs, 41–14, when Belichick, their famously media-hating coach, kept answering reporters' questions with four words: "We're on to Cincinnati." It was a message to his team and the world. He'd already moved past the embarrassing loss and was focused on the next hurdle. The 2–2 Patriots went on to finish the season 12–4 and to win the Super Bowl, their first in a decade.

It was time to move on to the other players in NECC's fraudulent enterprise. It would be another shot at history, at convicting a pharmacist whose drugs caused so much disease and injury.

On to Cincinnati. On to Glenn Chin.

Varghese and Strachan brought a similar murder case against Glenn Chin and got nearly the same result. A jury found Chin not guilty of the second-degree murders, but guilty of various other crimes.

Judge Stearns sentenced Cadden to nine years, Chin to eight.

Penny Laperriere, whose husband, Lyn, had died in Michigan, faced Cadden at his sentencing to give voice to the victims. "Since the night Mr. Cadden murdered my husband I find it difficult to sleep most nights," she said. She hadn't even been able to donate

Lyn's organs as he had wished because they were infected with mold.

Cadden issued a brief, tearful apology to Penny and other people in the courtroom whose lives NECC's drugs had shattered. Afterward, one meningitis victim told a newspaper reporter that he wished the judge would sentence Cadden to an injection of his contaminated methylpred. Dawn Elliott, an Indiana woman who survived fungal meningitis, was disheartened with the acquittals, especially given the jury's splits. "We were so close to getting murder charges," she said in an interview with WCVB-TV Boston.

Melanie Gomes, the juror who'd argued passionately to acquit Cadden of the murders, attended his sentencing, too. She felt terrible hearing Penny and the others' anguish. But it did not change her mind. She did not believe Cadden had meant to kill people. "He wasn't a mean person," she said two years later. He had been found guilty of appropriate charges, and she was satisfied that he would be going to prison.

Not all of the jurors felt the same way. The foreman, Hill, said that he had misunderstood the judge's instructions. "If it wasn't unanimous, it was not guilty," Hill told WBUR. Two other jurors, Dong Shin, the chef, and William Magalhaes said the same in interviews with local Boston media. They had supported guilty verdicts on murder but changed their votes to not guilty believing—incorrectly—that if they could not convince their whole cohort to convict, then they had to vote not guilty. Instead, the jury could have hung on twenty-one murders, giving the prosecution another shot. Now it was too late.

Neither man understood why Judge Stearns, after reading the split votes on the verdict form, had accepted it without inquiry. If the judge had known about the confusion, he could have ordered the jury to continue deliberations. But Stearns had made clear from the start that he never believed that a murder case was appropriate. "I do not find that the evidence established, or even came close to establishing . . . that [Cadden] acted with state of knowledge that a conviction for second-degree murder under relevant state law requires," he said before sentencing the pharmacist.

The acquittals closed the door. Varghese and Strachan could never retry Cadden for murder.

EPILOGUE

2019-2020: MORE THAN 100 DEAD, 793 CASES

NECC, FRAMINGHAM, MASSACHUSETTS

The building that once housed NECC's headquarters is now called ShopRecycled. Instead of gowned pharmacists, shelves of drugs, and autoclaves, the space is filled with ramshackle couches, shelves, and cabinets—furniture rescued from the recycling pile next door and prepped for resale.

The boxy brick building houses ghosts, too. A glove box—the aquarium-like contraption in which the pharmacists made drugs—occupies one corner, alongside a mountain of cardboard file storage boxes marked with the old company name. An employee working there said the building's owner, Greg Conigliaro, was required to keep records on-site for a few years due to the bankruptcy and other legal cases. Conigliaro faced up to five years in federal prison after a jury convicted him in 2018 of conspiracy to defraud the FDA. Judge Stearns later threw that conviction out, but an appeals court overturned him. The matter is still under appeal, but Conigliaro is running out of options.

DRACUT, MASSACHUSETTS

Budweiser in hand, Owen Finnegan sits on a barstool, music blaring through the dark sports bar.

He still does not know how the drugs were contaminated, exactly.

To Finnegan it doesn't matter. Doubt and guilt visit him when he closes his eyes at night. He had filled thousands of the vials with the contaminated lots of methylpred. He knows that he and his colleagues did things that compromised the safety of the products they made.

"I know it's stupid. This was a professional environment. An environment where sterility is of utmost importance. We're in there, and I'm guilty of this offense, wrestling around and slapping each other," he says between slugs of beer. "I'm not saying I'm not partly responsible. But again, that's the pharmacist's room. If [Glenn Chin or Barry Cadden] had a problem with it, nip it in the bud."

He finds himself, in slow moments at the collection agency where he now works, looking up news about the victims and how they're faring. "I torture myself by reading the articles. I read the Facebook posts of the victims and see things like 'I lost the use of a body part,' or 'I can't see.' It's just constant."

Finnegan wishes he'd never interviewed for the job at NECC.

ACROSS THE UNITED STATES

More than a hundred people have died from *Exserohilum rostratum* since being infected by NECC's methylprednisolone acetate, but hundreds more—some seven hundred across twenty states—live on. Carrie Mohr, forty-two, of Middlebury, Indiana, walks with a cane, eyes sallow, cheeks hollow. Mohr had been a veterinary technician, but working is impossible now. She was infected after her first round of steroid injections, and lives in constant pain with no idea when or if the fungus will resurface and take her life. Her surgeons have refused to operate to try to "clean out" the infected area. "What I have been told is introducing any foreign object into the area could reactivate the fungus."

Pills dictate every minute of Willard "J.R." Mazure's life in Pinconning, Michigan, a rural village on the shore of Saginaw Bay. The dirt-bike-racing, barn-building former construction worker survives on a constant rotation of antifungals, opiates, and other medications. Mazure earned a macabre milestone: he had the longest hospital stay—209 days—of any outbreak patient. He also believes he survived more doses of "amphoterrible" than anyone else. Now, seven back surgeries and $4 million in medical bills later, he still doesn't know if he's through it.

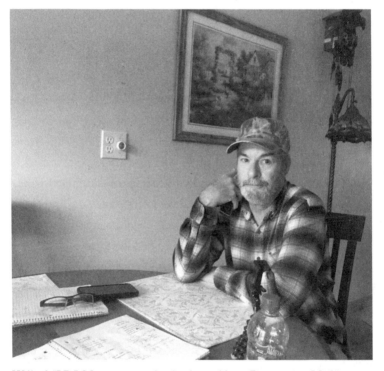

Willard "J.R." Mazure sits at his kitchen table in Pinconning, Michigan, in 2019. Mazure spent more than 200 days in the hospital after being injected with contaminated steroids produced by the New England Compounding Center. *(Courtesy of the author)*

In the Detroit suburb of New Hudson, Alan Przydzial became so verbally abusive toward his wife, Donna, that she left him. His personality had completely changed since being infected at age fifty-nine. When Al discovered that Donna was gone, he realized what he'd become: angry, reliant on pain meds for his throbbing back. His children helped enroll him in therapy, and after a few weeks, Al fell to his knees and begged Donna to come home. They are now living together again.

Many of NECC's victims were elderly people with chronic pain, but a significant number were middle-aged or younger. The youngest known victim was a sixteen-year-old, Zac Foutz of Virginia, who recovered enough to play college football and is now working on his master's degree in public health.

The CDC stopped officially tracking *Exserohilum rostratum* cases in October 2013, but conducted a long-term follow-up study of 440 patients to track how they were faring a year later. The findings, according to Dr. Tom Chiller of the CDC, one of the study's authors, found that a significant number of patients reported lingering effects. About 43 percent of patients who had fungal abscesses on their spines—like Mazure and Przydzial—remained on antifungals. They reported difficulty walking without assistance, and in some cases, worsening back pain. Eighty-seven percent of those respondents who survived had been cured, but most continued their lives in pain.

In the wake of the tragedy, hundreds of civil lawsuits were filed against NECC by victims, hospitals, and health insurers. The company filed for bankruptcy in December 2012, and most of the lawsuits were consolidated into one large case. Because there were so many suits and creditors, many of the victims have not been paid large settlements. Those who were awarded money have seen it greatly reduced as Medicare, Medicaid, and insurers sought reimbursement for unpaid hospital bills. After the victims' attorneys recouped their fees of 30 percent or more, most settlements to the victims themselves have been a pittance.

A separate $40 million victim's compensation fund set up by the federal government and administered by the state of Massachusetts paid claims capped at $25,000 or $50,000, depending on the case.

For some survivors and the family members of those who died, this is all the money they have yet to receive. While the court ordered Cadden to pay $82 million in restitution to the victims, it's unlikely they will see much, if any, of it.

THE WORLD

Dr. Benjamin Park and Dr. Rachel Smith of the CDC are still working together, but in a world changed by the COVID-19 pandemic. Park is chief of the International Infection Control Program, and led the group's efforts during the 2014 West Africa Ebola outbreak. He's now working to help the international communuity control the spread of COVID-19. He's also managed the CDC's efforts to help battle outbreaks of Middle East Respiratory Syndrome (MERS) in Saudi Arabia and Korea, as well as drug-resistant "superbugs" in Asia. Smith works for the same group as Park, leading a surveillance team that has investigated COVID-19, as well as illnesses caused by the fungus *Candida auris* in two hospitals in Panama, and a widespread measles outbreak in Ulaanbaatar, Mongolia.

Dr. Marion Kainer, the Tennessee epidemiologist whose quick thinking got the CDC's attention, testified in 2012 before Congress to warn about the dangers of unregulated compounded drugs. For her work alerting the nation about the outbreak and saving countless lives, she was honored with multiple awards, including being named Tennessee's Person of the Year by a Nashville newspaper. She recently moved back to her native Australia, where she serves as head of infectious diseases for a hospital group in Melbourne. Dr. April Pettit, who identified the first case of fungal meningitis in Tennessee, is an associate professor of medicine at Vanderbilt University Medical Center.

Beverly Jones, the Virginia biologist who first identified *Exserohilum rostratum* during the outbreak, still works in her small laboratory in Richmond. She's eyeing retirement now and looks forward to spending more time cycling, one of her passions other than fungi.

BOSTON

While George Varghese has gone into private practice, Amanda Strachan still works out of the U.S. Attorney's Office conference room with its view of the harbor. At one end hangs a U.S. flag, with the stars replaced with sixty-four hearts, one for each of the deaths known at that time, reading *Survivors* and *Don't Forget*—a gift from an outbreak victim. The flag reminds the prosecutors and myriad FBI and FDA agents who spent years poring through millions of documents why they were working so hard. Strachan is now chief of the Health Care Fraud Unit. Her office still works on NECC-related cases.

Ultimately, the federal government convicted thirteen people on 178 charges. Strachan and Varghese sometimes feel the murder acquittals were a failure of the justice system. Judge Richard G. Stearns was openly skeptical of the government's case, which he deemed bloated. The prosecutors and many of the meningitis survivors also fault him for not sending the jury back to deliberate after he saw the split-vote totals that could have led to a hung jury and a second chance for the prosecution.

"I feel like the health care system in this country really failed the victims. And then the justice system really failed them. And it just made me so sad to be a part of the latter," Strachan reflected recently.

HOWELL, MICHIGAN

Barry Cadden and Glenn Chin received initial federal prison sentences of nine and eight years, respectively. However, in 2021 the court increased Cadden's sentence to fourteen and a half years. A federal appeals court ruled that Judge Stearns had improperly calculated the initial sentence. Chin's was also increased. NECC's majority owners Dr. Douglas Conigliaro and his wife, Carla, were convicted of charges related to the transferring of millions of dollars illegally after the outbreak occurred. Federal officials seized nearly $17 million from the couple's accounts. They received probation and $60,000 in fines. A handful of other NECC pharmacists have faced a jury and earned short prison terms or probation.

Cadden's lead attorneys, Bruce Singal and Michelle Peirce, continue to represent him. In November 2019, Singal stood before a panel of three federal judges in Boston to argue that Cadden's convictions should be thrown out on appeal. Holding on to the podium, Singal railed against the prosecution's use of "grisly and emotional" evidence. Health care cases in Boston have become Singal's bread and butter, and that of the firm he co-chairs, Barrett & Singal.

It's possible that Barrett & Singal will be defending Cadden for years to come. Michigan, the state hardest hit by the outbreak with at least twenty-three related deaths, has filed more second-degree murder charges against Cadden and Glenn Chin. Both pharmacists are likely to be back in court facing life sentences.

THE STATE OF COMPOUNDING

In 2016, nurses in the pediatric units of hospitals in Chicago and Indianapolis administered a pain medication, morphine sulfate, to an unknown number of infants. Three immediately suffered overdoses. One had to be revived using Narcan, an opioid overdose treatment, and airlifted to a neonatal intensive care unit at another hospital. All three barely survived.

The FDA learned that both hospitals received the drugs from a compounding pharmacy called Pharmakon Pharmaceuticals. Further investigation uncovered that the drugs were 2,460 percent too potent. When FDA inspectors checked the pharmacy's records, they learned that its then president, Paul Elmer, and its compliance director, Caprice Bearden, regularly covered up evidence of multiple potency failures.

FDA inspectors had long known that Pharmakon posed a risk. Two years before the infant overdoses the agency learned that it distributed a sedative called midazolam, used to treat premature infants at a hospital in Indianapolis, that was 200 percent too strong. The FDA inspected Pharmakon but did not shut them down. The agency later said that Elmer and Bearden hid the evidence of their cover-ups from inspectors. The Pharmakon drugs that caused these infant overdoses were among more than seventy batches of untested compounded medicines sent to U.S. hospitals by just this one company.

No one knows how many patient deaths and injuries occur each year due to errors in compounding drugs. Compounders are not required to report these overdoses in the FDA's database of adverse events caused by pharmaceuticals. This lack of mandatory reporting was a key victory for the compounding industry in the fight to weaken 2013's Drug Quality and Security Act (DQSA)—the federal law passed in response to the NECC outbreak. An effort by the Pew Charitable Trusts to quantify these deaths and injuries anecdotally found 1,418 adverse events and 114 deaths between 2001 and 2017. Pew cautioned that that number is probably a drop in the bucket: the NECC outbreak alone killed more than 100 patients and sickened nearly 800 others.

Since the DQSA's passage, evidence of hundreds of adverse events from compounded drugs has surfaced. In 2013, as Congress debated the DQSA, fifteen patients in Texas developed bacterial bloodstream infections, and another two died, after receiving IV medications from an outfit named Specialty Compounding. In 2016, seventeen people in New York contracted fungal blood infections, and at least two died, at an outpatient cancer clinic that gave people contaminated intravenous solutions compounded on-site. In

2017, forty-one patients in New Jersey were diagnosed with septic arthritis after receiving bacteria-contaminated injections. The investigation found substandard aseptic technique in the clinics' own compounding areas where the bulk packaged drug was improperly separated into individual doses.

In 2017, during cataract surgeries and other procedures, surgeons at the Key-Whitman Eye Center in Dallas injected a drug called Tri-Moxi into their patients' eyes. It was supposed to stop swelling, infection, and dryness. It instead blinded and visually impaired at least forty-three people. The Tri-Moxi was made at Guardian Pharmacy Services, a drug compounder that had not voluntarily registered with the FDA under the DQSA. For a time, Key-Whitman had purchased its Tri-Moxi from one of the FDA-approved "outsourcing facilities," a category created by the law, but the clinic switched temporarily to Guardian's cheaper product.

Guardian's owner, Jack Munn, sold the medication to the eye surgery center even though his pharmacy had no previous experience making it. Instead of volunteering to develop an unfamiliar product under the eye of the FDA, he called the Professional Compounding Centers of America (PCCA) for help. Guardian then compounded what authorities would later call a "seriously flawed" drug. A review of Guardian's prior run-ins with regulators found similar warning signs as those for NECC. Guardian shipped drugs without proper testing or valid prescriptions, and it had to recall drugs in 2016 and 2017 after inspectors found unsanitary conditions. In legal filings, Munn denied that his drugs caused the patients' problems and blamed it on a bad recipe from PCCA. PCCA pointed the finger back at Munn.

The DQSA failed to require the compounding pharmacy industry to report how many drugs they make. Neither the FDA nor most states has any clue. However, there is some evidence that the use of compounded medications continues to skyrocket. Medicare

Part D spending on compounded medications increased from $70.2 million in 2006 to $508.7 million in 2015. Government Accountability Office investigators located data from a single unidentified state that reported 708,142 prescriptions and almost two million units of sterile drugs were distributed by pharmacies in 2015. Larger states like Texas told the GAO's investigators that "because they have thousands of licensed pharmacies in their state, the volume of such data would be overwhelming and they do not know what they would do with all of that data."

Meanwhile, hospitals—such as the two in Chicago and Indiana whose morphine sulfate sickened infants in the pediatric unit—are still giving patients non-FDA-approved compounded drugs with no labels. The DQSA has increased the number of compounding pharmacies that volunteer for FDA oversight, providing hospitals with a route to obtain safer drugs. But there are major cracks in this discretionary federal system: namely, only seventy-six of the thousands of sterile compounding pharmacies estimated to be operating in the United States have joined. The bill's supporters on Capitol Hill believed this pool of FDA-approved "outsourcing facilities" would become a lucrative market. But the pharmacies that have registered are subject to a frustrating tangle of rules that limits their output, and they must invest in expensive upgrades to comply with the agency's Current Good Manufacturing Practices. Complicating matters further, as of the writing of this book the FDA had yet to approve its list of the bulk active pharmaceutical ingredients that these outsourcers could legally use to make drugs without prescriptions.

An internal Department of Health and Human Services audit, details of which the author obtained using the Freedom of Information Act, determined that at least 11 percent of the some six hundred hospitals it surveyed were still buying drugs from non-FDA-registered facilities. (Because the OIG's questionnaire was

voluntary, the actual number is likely much higher.) It also identified forty unregistered compounding pharmacies in twenty-two
states that are selling directly to hospitals without patient-specific
prescriptions. According to FDA records, some have been recently
cited by agency inspectors for "serious deficiencies" in their handling of sterile drugs. Despite this obvious red alert, these compounders are still selling medications made in substandard
conditions to hospitals.

The DQSA also sought to limit the amount of compounded
drugs shipped between states without prescriptions—initially set at
5 percent, unless the states signed a Memorandum of Understanding with the FDA. But because this data is not tracked, this limit
is impossible to enforce. It was meant to limit the flow of compounded drugs bought by doctors for "office use," which they can
legally give patients without prescriptions in emergencies. Compounders immediately threatened to sue, and the FDA, cowed by
the thought of unceasing litigation from the IACP/Alliance for
Pharmacy Compounding's members in each state, agreed not to
enforce the limit. Regardless, if neither the FDA nor the state
boards of pharmacy track the number of drugs produced or shipped
into their state from outside, how can they possibly know if a pharmacy exceeds the 5 percent ceiling?

State boards, the sole watchdogs of most compounders in the U.S.,
do not have the money or bodies to conduct inspections, especially
when pharmacies are in another state. A move toward an accreditation for compounding pharmacies via the National Association of
Boards of Pharmacy—an umbrella group of state regulators—may
help, but it is voluntary.

With no fix on the horizon, the DQSA's modest safety gains remain under assault from some of the same lawmakers who resisted
FDA oversight during the NECC outbreak. Republican congressman Morgan Griffith of Virginia, a longtime ally and cash recipi-

ent of the compounding industry, has sponsored multiple bills since 2013 seeking to make compounding easier. His bills have sought to legalize the use of non-FDA-approved dietary supplements in compounded drugs. Another would remove any limits on the quantities of compounded medicines that can be shipped between states. So far, none of Griffith's bills have made it out of any Congressional committee.

Just as before the outbreak, states are still responsible for ensuring the safety of the vast majority of compounded drugs. Some states have passed tougher rules in the years since. Out of thirty-nine compounding pharmacies that Massachusetts inspectors checked in 2012–2013, only four passed inspection. Eleven received full or partial cease and desist orders because they posed an immediate threat to public safety. Michigan, California, Texas, and other states are also monitoring the industry more closely. Some states have also allowed the FDA to inspect more large compounders, improving safety at those facilities.

Still, a 2016–2017 Government Accountability Office study described a piecemeal system riddled with lapses. Sterile drugs are being made in a variety of conditions by pharmacists and non-pharmacists alike. Pharmacy boards in eighteen states remain confused about the proper settings in which sterile drugs can be legally compounded in their jurisdictions.

The COVID-19 pandemic has further confused oversight of compounding pharmacies. In 2020, the FDA relaxed the agency's guidelines for compounding so pharmacists could make more drugs to help with hospital shortages. Industry lobbyists are working to make FDA's emergency COVID-19 rules permanent, setting up another political battle over lax oversight of companies like NECC that are shipping injectable drugs over state lines.

And legal troubles loom for one of the compounding industry's foundational companies, PCCA, the Professional Compounding

Centers of America, Inc. In November 2021, the U.S. Department of Justice filed a fraud case alleging price inflation and other charges. The complaint further alleges that PCCA knew it was selling and promoting drug formulations that were potentially harmful. The company has denied all the allegations and said it is primed to fight. But the DOJ's action against one of the industry's key suppliers shows concerns about the industry have risen to the highest levels of the federal government.

Sarah Sellers, the pharmacist and former FDA compounding safety expert, said that in the wake of the fungal meningitis outbreak, the FDA and state boards asked for a simpler, clearer mandate to better ensure a safe supply of drugs. What it got was the DQSA, which she sees as a Gordian knot. The laws are now *more* complicated and easier to exploit. "You better be damn careful when you're going to exempt drugs from the Food, Drug, and Cosmetic Act, and we're not being damn careful. This is ridiculously cavalier."

WHAT TO ASK YOUR PRESCRIBER ABOUT COMPOUNDED DRUGS

Since the 1990s there has been a resurgence in the practice of pharmacy compounding in the United States. While there is no definitive source to educate patients about exactly how much of the country's drug supply is made by pharmacy compounding, a safe guess based on limited data is at least 10 percent.

Most compounding pharmacies are still not held to the same high safety rules as drug manufacturers, so drug quality can vary widely. It is important to ask questions of your doctors and pharmacists. A good rule of thumb is that if a drug is being injected, it's wise to be more cautious.

Rita Weiss is a pharmacist (RPh, CPh) and attorney who inspects compounding pharmacies as an onsite surveyor/inspector for the National Association of Boards of Pharmacy.

Weiss believes patients should ask the following questions of their prescriber, especially before any surgical procedures:

1. Will I be receiving a compounded medication during the procedure, or will you be prescribing me a compounded medication?

2. If the answer is yes, why are you using and/or prescribing a compounded medication?

Good reasons:

   a. The drug is not made by a drug manufacturer. If this is the answer, ask:

      i. Why is it not made by a manufacturer?

ii. Why do you believe that there are no drugs made by a manufacturer that will work in the same way that the compounded medication will work?

iii. Is the compounding pharmacy that is making the drug product registered with the FDA?

- How do you know it is registered?

- When was the last time you checked that the FDA registration is current?

- Do you know if the compounding pharmacy has been inspected by the FDA, and if it has, did it receive a 483 (warning letter), and did the company respond?

b. The drug is normally made by a drug manufacturer, but there is a shortage. If this is the answer, ask:

i. Do you know when the shortage started and why there is a shortage?

ii. Would it be a safe course of action for me to wait to have the procedure done until the commercially available product is available?

iii. Is there a commercially available product available that can be prescribed instead, and will it provide similar results?

c. The prescriber believes that a compounded medication is a better choice for you. If this is the answer, ask:

i. What does the compounded medication offer that a commercially available product does not?

ii. Are you directing me to use only one compounding pharmacy to obtain the prescription? *If the prescriber insists on sending the prescription to only one compounding pharmacy, you should refuse and seek treatment elsewhere.*

If your doctor gives any of the following reasons for prescribing you a compounded drug, you should investigate the issue further and/or get a second opinion:

a. The compounded medication is cheaper from a compounding pharmacy.

b. The compounded medication has a longer shelf life or expiration date than the commercially available product.

c. The compounded medication is available overseas, but not in the United States. If this is the case, ask why it is not available as a commercial product in the United States.

d. The compounded medication will give you better results. Ask why.

3. Does the compounding pharmacy require that you provide my allergy information, current medication therapy information, and current disease state information, to screen for contraindications before compounding for me?

4. Is the compounding pharmacy regularly inspected by the state board of pharmacy? Do you know when it was last inspected, and do you have a copy of the inspection report?

5. Has the state board of pharmacy ever sanctioned or otherwise disciplined the pharmacy or the pharmacists who work in the pharmacy? If so, do you know why?

6. Does the compounding pharmacy have any type of national accreditation, and if so, is it current and in good standing?

7. If the compounding pharmacy is not located in your state, does it have an out-of-state license to ship into your state?

8. Does the pharmacy compound in batches? In other words, does it mix ingredients to create a compounded medication in quantities large enough to fill the prescription for more than one patient? If yes, how are the batches tested?

a. If the medication in question is a sterile product, is the batch tested according to USP guidelines?

b. Is the lab that does the test independently owned and operated, separate from the pharmacy?

9. Have you ever received a recall notice from the compounding pharmacy? If yes, ask more about why the product was recalled and who initiated the recall (the pharmacy or a government entity).

10. Do you, or a friend or family member, have a monetary interest in the compounding pharmacy?

ACKNOWLEDGMENTS

In August 2001, I moved to Manhattan to attend graduate school. Weeks later the World Trade Center fell to ashes. Reporting became my lodestar and obsession. Two professors at Columbia University's Graduate School of Journalism, Sig Gissler and Samuel G. Freedman, gave me invaluable tools and encouragement—in the school's basic reporting class and later in Freedman's nonfiction book seminar. I came away from these classes fully aware of my shortcomings, but also with a clear sense of the hard work it takes to produce the kind of journalism I admire.

Reporting is a team sport, and I've learned from some of the best in the business: my colleagues at the Associated Press. I want to give a special thanks to former AP features editor Pauline Arrillaga, who encouraged me to look into the fungal meningitis outbreak. Also, thanks to Brian Carovillano, Tim Reiterman, Garance Burke, and countless others who helped me out along the way.

Of course, this book would not have been possible without access to key sources including the victims and their families, the U.S. Attorney's Office in Boston, the U.S. Centers for Disease Control and Prevention in Atlanta, the staff at St. Joseph Mercy Hospital in Ann Arbor, numerous state public health departments, health care policy analysts in both the U.S. Senate and House of Representatives and at the Pew Charitable Trusts, and current and former staff at the U.S. Food and Drug Administration. They all believed this was an important story and donated significant time.

Nonfiction requires a lot of source material. I got thousands of pages of notes and documents, thanks to the work of federal prosecutors Amanda Strachan and George Varghese, who also sat patiently for days of interviews. The NECC victims opened their homes and shared their stories:

Willard and Linda Mazure; Alan and Donna Przydzial; the Lovelace and Talbott families; Penny Laperriere; Pamela Kidd; Anna Allred; Carrie Mohr; and Ray Gipson.

At the CDC, Dr. Benjamin Park, Dr. Rachel Smith, Dr. Mary Brandt, and Dr. Sherif Zaki gave me significant time. Others at the agency who provided important help: Dr. Tom Chiller, Dr. Ray Dantes, Dr. J. Todd Weber, and Dave Daigle. I could not have written this book without Dr. Marion Kainer at the Tennessee Department of Health and, at Vanderbilt University Medical Center, Dr. April Pettit and mycology lab technician Tonya Snyder. In Ann Arbor, St. Joe's communications director Laura Blodgett, Dr. Anurag Malani, and Dr. Varsha Moudgal. At the Michigan Department of Health and Human Services: Lynn Sutfin, Jim Collins, Jay Fiedler, and Jim Coyle. At Virginia's Department of General Services: Dena Potter and Beverly Jones. Former New England Compounding Center pharmacy technician Owen Finnegan spent hours in person, over email, and by phone answering every question I asked.

In Washington, I am thankful to the current and former Capitol Hill and U.S. Food and Drug Administration staffers, lobbyists, and policy experts who helped me tell the story of the Drug Quality and Security Act. Most requested that their names not be used, but I am especially grateful to the die-hard Sarah Sellers, who dug out hundreds of old records and spent hours helping me understand the unsuccessful efforts to regulate this fast-growing industry. Also a special thanks to Jennifer Boyer and current and former Senate HELP Committee staffers who revealed to me how the sausage was made.

My kind and hardworking agent, Danielle Svetcov, at the Levine Greenberg Rostan Literary Agency, was a foundation for me during the three years I worked on this book. Danielle guided me through the publishing world and edited drafts of each chapter. Thanks, too, to my friend James Nestor for introducing me to Danielle, and for his critical reading.

Avery Books publisher Megan Newman took a chance on a first-time author. My editor, Nina Shield, did what the best editors do: she saved me from myself (any overwrought passages are mine alone). Also thanks to the wonderful copyeditor, Nancy Inglis, for her careful reading. Thanks, Megan, Nina, and the entire Avery–Penguin Random House team.

I conducted much of the early research as a Knight Science Journalism Fellow at MIT. It was a dream year, thanks to Deborah Blum, Ashley Smart, Bettina Urcuioli, Pakinam Amer, Magnus Bjerg, Talia Bronstein, Lisa De Bode, Tim De Chant, Jeffery DelViscio, Elana Gordon, and Amina Khan. Special thanks to fellow Knight Rachel Gross, who took time away from her own book to help me.

All hail librarians! Especially Alison P. Kelly at the Library of Congress; Danielle Castronovo at the Harvard Botany Libraries; and Harvard's Dr. Donald Pfister, curator of the Farlow Library and Herbarium of Cryptogamic Botany. The Alfred P. Sloan Foundation's Public Understanding of Science book grant and its director, Doron Weber, provided critical support that allowed me to hire a fact checker, Kelsey Kudak. Kelsey improved the book immensely and dug deep into the weeds with me. Any remaining errors are my fault. Thanks also to my science reviewers, Dr. Roger Shapiro and Dr. Rita Weiss.

Finally, thanks to my wife, Stephanie Bornstein. She read the rawest drafts of each chapter and gave me the most important feedback any writer could hope for: the truth, with a heavy sigh, no matter what. Steph, there's no one with whom I'd rather be in the trenches.

NOTES

PROLOGUE

xi **The seventy-eight-year-old still walked three miles every morning:**
Scenes from Eddie Lovelace's final days and his funeral were
reconstructed from a reporting trip by the author to Lovelace's home in
Albany, Kentucky; interviews with his wife, Joyce Lovelace; his daughter,
Karen Talbott; and other family members. The author also obtained a
copy of his autopsy report, visited the cemetery where Lovelace's body
was exhumed and reburied, and interviewed other friends and relatives.

CHAPTER 1. PATIENT ZERO

1 **the fifty-five-year-old father of three:** The opening scene of Tom and
Collette Rybinski's lake trip in Tennessee was constructed from Collette's
courtroom testimony during the Barry Cadden trial as well as excerpts of
her secret grand jury testimony obtained by the author. The author also
interviewed state and federal epidemiologists at the Centers for Disease
Control and Prevention and the Tennessee Department of Health about
Rybinski's case, and visited the Vanderbilt University Medical Center hospital
room where Rybinski was treated in order to obtain descriptive details.

3 **Thomas Rybinski was a man in his fifties:** Scenes of Dr. April Pettit's
interactions with Tom Rybinski and his family at Vanderbilt University
Medical Center were built through multiple interviews with Dr. Pettit
and her colleagues, a reporting trip by the author to the hospital, and
Collette Rybinski's courtroom testimony.

4 **Six days after Rybinski was readmitted:** Clinical details from Tom
Rybinski's case were published in a scientific paper: Dr. April C. Pettit
et al., "The Index Case for the Fungal Meningitis Outbreak in the United
States," *New England Journal of Medicine* 367 (2012): 2119–25.

7   **Pettit's email set off alarm bells**: Marion Kainer's scenes were developed
     from multiple interviews with her in Tennessee, copies of emails she sent
     and received during the outbreak, reports she wrote about her
     methodology and management of the unfolding crisis, and interviews
     with her colleagues at the Tennessee Department of Public Health.

11   **In Atlanta, Park began digging around**: Scenes at the CDC were
     built using internal agency records and emails, a number of interviews
     with Dr. Ben Park and a dozen of his colleagues during multiple
     visits to CDC's Atlanta campus, and published case studies of the
     epidemiological response to the outbreak: Dr. Marion Kainer et al.,
     "Fungal Infections Associated with Contaminated Methylprednisolone
     in Tennessee," *New England Journal of Medicine* 367 (2012): 2194–2203.

CHAPTER 2. THE FERRARI OF COMPOUNDERS

13   **Barry Cadden leaned forward**: The scene that runs throughout the
     chapter of Barry Cadden's addressing his sales force was built from
     hours of videotapes of his sales seminars and notes taken by attendees
     that were seized by the U.S. government during its criminal investigation
     of the New England Compounding Center. The author obtained copies
     of the videos and notes from the U.S. Attorney's Office in Boston.

14   **There were many reasons for the shortfalls**: C. Lee Ventola, "The Drug
     Shortage Crisis in the United States," *Pharmacy & Therapeutics* 2011 Nov;
     36(11): 740–42, 749–57.

17   **As he let go of existing employees**: This description of the NECC sales
     department as a "cutthroat atmosphere" comes from former sales rep
     Kenneth Boneau, who testified during the criminal trial against
     pharmacist Glenn Chin.

17   **Watching over the group was national sales director Rob Ronzio**:
     Robert Ronzio refused to be interviewed for this book. I attended his
     trial testimony during the later NECC trial for Gregory Conigliaro and
     four other defendants, and used transcripts of his testimony during the
     Cadden and Chin trials to build scenes with Ronzio. I also had access to
     dozes of his emails that were presented as evidence during the NECC
     criminal trials. I also spoke with the federal prosecutors who interviewed
     him as a witness, as well as his former colleagues at NECC.

20   **Sending out drugs without patient prescriptions is illegal**: Information
     about the problems plaguing the Massachusetts Board of Registration in
     Pharmacy came from the testimony of its lead inspector, Samuel Penta,

in the Barry Cadden and Glenn Chin trials; from the agency's documents published during the trials; and the findings of an investigative report by the U.S. House of Representatives published in the aftermath of the outbreak, *FDA'S Oversight of NECC and Ameridose: A History of Missed Opportunities?* (2013).

21 Before the U.S. Pharmacopeia changed its safety standards: NECC's sales figures were compiled by the FBI and the U.S. Attorney's Office and were included in a slideshow prosecutors displayed during the trial.

22 Cadden's predilection to skirt safeguards: The information about NECC's previous adverse events came from court documents, FDA inspection reports, and the U.S. House of Representatives' *Missed Opportunities* investigative report.

24 Listening to Cadden: Reactions to Cadden's sales talks came from the handwritten notes and testimony of two salesmen who attended, Ken Boneau and Mario Giamei, during Barry Cadden's criminal trial, and interviews with other former employees.

24 Mario Giamei looked like a bouncer: Information about Giamei was derived from his testimony during the Cadden and Chin trials, and I attended his testimony during a third, related trial in Boston. I also obtained dozens of emails he sent during the outbreak. Information for this section also came from interviews with the assistant U.S. attorneys George Varghese and Amanda Strachan, a doctor and NECC client in Tennessee, and a coworker. Giamei declined to be interviewed for this book.

30 It wasn't always seamless: Evidence of NECC clients who asked questions about its policies and procedures, yet who kept purchasing drugs from them, came from company emails presented during the Cadden and Chin criminal trials.

CHAPTER 3. A SLOW-MOVING MASS-CASUALTY EVENT

33 Dr. John Culclasure felt like crying: This scene with Dr. John Culclasure was built through his testimony at the Cadden and Chin criminal trials, interviews, a visit to the St. Thomas Outpatient Neurosurgical Center in Tennessee, and court documents that included emails sent between Culclasure and NECC.

34 When Culclasure walked into the procedure room: Culclasure detailed each step of his process for an epidural steroid injection during testimony in the Cadden and Chin trials.

35 **Giamei arrived at the St. Thomas clinic:** The scene between Dr. John
    Culclasure, his nurse Debra Schamberg, and NECC salesman Mario
    Giamei was built through their testimony at the Cadden and Chin
    criminal trials, interviews, a visit to the St. Thomas Outpatient
    Neurosurgical Center in Tennessee, and court documents that included
    emails sent between Culclasure's staff and NECC.

37 **"It's us," Cadden said:** This scene and Cadden's quotes come from Rob
    Ronzio's testimony in the Cadden trial, as well as the testimony of FBI
    special agent Philip Sliney.

38 **For nearly two decades Jones had served:** Scenes from Beverly Jones's
    Virginia lab were built based on documents provided by the Virginia
    Department of Health, interviews with Jones at her lab in Richmond and
    with the CDC's Dr. Mary Brandt.

39 **Dr. Ben Park huddled before a speakerphone:** The scene of this
    important first call with Barry Cadden and others at NECC was built
    from interviews with Dr. Ben Park and Dr. Rachel Smith of the CDC,
    Dr. Smith's notes of the call, trial testimony, and interviews with Dr.
    Marion Kainer of the Tennessee Department of Public Health.

40 **This early version of the CDC:** The history of the CDC was taken from
    the agency's website and the book *Beating Back the Devil* by Maryn
    McKenna (New York: Free Press, 2008).

44 **Effie Elwina Shaw lay:** Details of Elwina Shaw's case come from
    interviews with Dr. Ben Park and Dr. Rachel Smith at the CDC,
    interviews with Shaw's daughter Anna Allred, and Allred's testimony in
    the Barry Cadden trial.

46 **Forty-eight hours had elapsed:** This scene was built from multiple
    interviews with Dr. Rachel Smith and Dr. Ben Park, internal CDC
    emails, handwritten notes of the call taken by Dr. Smith, and visits to
    the CDC.

CHAPTER 4. BULLETPROOF

53 **Inside a concrete hospital tower:** Details of the Massachusetts Eye and
    Ear case of sub-potent drugs made by NECC came from the testimony
    and emails of the hospital's chief pharmacist, Jo Stewart, and other Mass.
    Eye employees who testified in the Barry Cadden trial.

56 **Owen Finnegan pulled into the parking lot:** Scene details inside
    NECC's clean room are based on interviews with Owen Finnegan in
    person and by phone, as well as testimony from him and other NECC

pharmacy technicians who testified during the three main NECC criminal trials. I also used emails from staff and the logged formula worksheets they created when compounding batches of drugs, which were presented as evidence during the NECC criminal trials. To get a sense of what it felt like inside a clean room, I also visited one at the University of Florida's Cancer Hospital in Gainesville, Florida.

56   **The next day, Connolly received:** Copies of this specific logged formula worksheet were presented as evidence at trial, and Connolly testified about the incident in detail under oath.

57   **The majority owner:** Details of the family's finances and real estate holdings come from court documents and a *New York Times* story: Abby Goodnough, Sabrina Tavernise, and Andrew Pollack, "Spotlight Put on Founders of Drug Firm in Outbreak," *New York Times*, October 24, 2012.

57   **"The lab downstairs is the engine":** This email from Barry Cadden was obtained from the evidence presented during his murder trial.

58   **"Just beginning to scratch surface":** Scans of Cadden's handwritten notes were included in the evidence presented during his murder trial.

59   **Parts of the room's shiny, pale green floors:** Numerous NECC pharmacy technicians including Owen Finnegan and Joe Connolly testified about the cracks in the floor and the oily substance oozing through. NECC was built atop a hazardous waste site, a spot where there had been a significant oil spill years earlier. This was confirmed through county records, and I even obtained a map of the oil spill's footprint, showing that it covered much of the building area where NECC built its clean room.

60   **Early mornings in the lab:** Testimony by NECC pharmacy technicians Owen Finnegan, Joseph Connolly, and others confirmed the constant presence of insects and mice in the NECC building. I also obtained emails from head pharmacist Glenn Chin referring to flies and other bugs in the trial exhibits.

62   **Chin made sure to remind him:** This quote from Glenn Chin comes from Owen Finnegan's testimony under oath in the Cadden trial and was confirmed during an in-person interview.

63   **Chin pulled the male employees aside:** Details from the testimony of NECC pharmacy technician Owen Finnegan, his interviews with me, and court documents filed by Tucker against NECC.

63   **Humans are host to trillions of microscopic residents:** Details about the struggles to contain contamination from workers in a clean room come from Charles E. Myers, "History of Sterile Compounding in U.S.

Hospitals: Learning from the Tragic Lessons of the Past," *American Journal of Health-System Pharmacy* 70, no. 16 (August 15, 2013): 1414–27.

67   **On July 5, she found woolly "overgrown mold":** Annette Robinson's testing logs were included as evidence exhibits in the Barry Cadden and Glenn Chin trials, and were obtained by the author.

69   **But Cadden neither sent the testing data nor agreed to the antifungal cleaning:** Details of Barry Cadden's failure to follow up on his cleaning company's offers to bomb the clean room with antifungal agent comes from the testimony of UniClean's Edwin Cardona, the company's contamination control manager, as well as emails between the two presented as evidence during Cadden's criminal trial.

CHAPTER 5. SHADOW INDUSTRY

71   **When Letson came onstage:** This scene of Mickey Letson's speech about the rising fortunes of the compounding industry was built off a transcript of the speech.

72   **Behind the scenes, the FDA's staff:** Comments about the state of the FDA's early efforts to regulate pharmacy compounding come from interviews with current and former employees who requested anonymity, and the public testimony of FDA officials following the fungal meningitis outbreak.

76   **In 1857, a story in *The New York Times*:** "The Late Fatal Mistake in Baltimore," *New York Times,* January 27, 1857.

76   **In 1893, a young drug clerk:** "Gave Morphine by Mistake," *New York Times,* January 11, 1893.

77   **One of the resulting inspection reports:** *Treasury Department Digest of Comments on the Pharmacopoeia of the USA and on the National Formulary,* U.S. Library of Congress (1921).

77   **Watkins had developed a raspberry-flavored syrup:** Information about the Elixir Sulfanilamide poisonings came from a feature on the incident published by the U.S. FDA.

78   **Commercial production of so-called wonder drugs:** Details about the mid-twentieth-century's drug manufacturing boom were taken from the fascinating book *Medicating Modern America: Prescription Drugs in History,* by Andrea Tone and Elizabeth Siegel Watkins (New York: New York University Press, 2007).

78 **By the early 1980s, only 2 percent of all prescriptions:** Mickey Smith and David Knapp, *Pharmacy, Drugs, and Medical Care* (New York: Williams & Wilkins, 1981), 62.

80 **Plus, as compounding pharmacies proliferated:** Details about pressures on FDA inspectors in the 2000s because of the foreign generic drug boom comes from Katherine Eban's *Bottle of Lies: The Inside Story of the Generic Drug Boom* (New York: Ecco, 2019).

80 **By 2010, at least 10 percent:** While no one truly knows the actual percentage of drugs compounded in the United States, this is the best estimate I could find. It came from an evidentiary stipulation in the Gregory Conigliaro trial, written by U.S. District Judge Richard Stearns: "The compounding industry is growing. Studies estimate that less than 1 percent of all prescriptions were compounded in the 1970s; that figure was expected to grow to 10 percent by 2010."

81 **When the FDA's compounding safety committee dissolved:** Details of Sarah Sellers's life and career in drug safety were taken from multiple interviews at her home in the Chicago area, as well as emails, documents, and videos of her testimony before the U.S. Senate's HELP Committee.

81 **In 2002, another compounding-related death:** Details of this case of death caused by a contaminated drug from a compounding pharmacy was included in the testimony of Dr. Janet Woodcock, director of the Center for Drug Evaluation and Research at the U.S. FDA, before the Senate HELP Committee in 2013.

82 **In 2001, it determined that 34 percent:** "FDA: Report: Limited FDA Survey of Compounded Drug Products," https://www.fda.gov/drugs /human-drug-compounding/report-limited-fda-survey-compounded -drug-products.

82 **"We have received reports":** Details from this 2003 hearing about the safety of compounded drugs was taken from video and transcripts provided by C-SPAN and the U.S. Senate.

85 **Within months she was pulled from the compounding working group:** Details of Sarah Sellers's tenure at the FDA came from interviews with her and from emails obtained by the author, and were confirmed by a retired FDA official who worked with Sellers at the time.

CHAPTER 6. SIX CONFOUNDING CASES

87 **Lyn Laperriere sat in his bed:** Details of Lyn's case come from interviews with his wife Penny Laperriere, interviews with doctors at

St. Joseph Mercy Hospital in Ann Arbor, the testimony of his pathologist in the Cadden criminal trial, and medical records.

88   **The head of the infectious disease department:** Scenes from St. Joseph Mercy Hospital came from multiple interviews with Dr. Varsha Moudgal, Dr. Anurag Malani, and other hospital staff, including surgeons, pharmacists, radiologists, lab staff, and others. I also met with multiple fungal meningitis survivors throughout Michigan who were treated at St. Joe's and with the loved ones of patients who died. The hospital also provided me with records and a timeline of the outbreak.

89   **Day 15, October 2, 2012: 2 dead, 14 cases:** Numbers reported by Joe Sutton of CNN in the article "Tennessee: Meningitis Outbreak Is Investigated," https://www.cnn.com/2012/10/02/health/tennessee -meningitis-outbreak/index.html.

90   **Chatas injected the steroid into his brother's neck:** Details of Dr. Chatas's injecting his brother were included in his colleague Dr. Edward Washabaugh's testimony at the Cadden trial, and elements of the case were confirmed by the author through interviews with hospital staff at St. Joseph Mercy Hospital in Ann Arbor and Michigan's state public health department.

90   *The New York Times* **ran its first story:** Denise Grady, "Meningitis Cases Are Linked to Steroid Injections in Spine," *New York Times*, October 2, 2012.

CHAPTER 7. A HOUSE OF CARDS

93   **The morning before his call with Ben Park and Marion Kainer:** Details about Barry Cadden's state of mind and his moves during the first few days of the fungal meningitis outbreak were built from court documents, including the emails he sent. I also relied on interviews with former NECC employees like Owen Finnegan, as well as the testimony of pharmacy tech Joseph Connolly and NECC sales director Robert Ronzio.

94   **On the call with the CDC, Cadden projected:** The details of this call and of Barry Cadden's demeanor came from multiple sources who participated: Dr. Ben Park and Dr. Rachel Smith at CDC, and Dr. Marion Kainer at the Tennessee Department of Public Health. Dr. Smith had taken handwritten notes of the call and shared them with me.

94   **As Cadden prepared, a nurse at a clinic:** This email from September 25, 2012, was among those included in the criminal trial exhibits and was

used by prosecutors during Cadden's federal criminal trial to argue that he was not telling NECC customers the truth, at a key moment in the outbreak, about the level of danger they faced.

94 **The evidence was increasingly pointing:** This email from September 25, 2012, was among hundreds obtained by the author and included as evidence in Cadden's federal criminal trial.

94 **On September 26 at 2:18 A.M., Cadden started calling:** Cadden's phone calls were included in transcripts of his murder trial. The defense introduced them as evidence that he was trying to alert as many customers as possible to the recall of the contaminated lots of steroids.

95 **Flanked by his three colleagues:** Details of the Massachusetts Board of Regulation in Pharmacy's initial inspection of NECC during the early days of the fungal meningitis outbreak came from the testimony of the lead inspector, Sam Penta, during multiple NECC criminal trials, his written reports, and emails between the board and NECC.

97 **They were in over their heads:** The board's decision to ask for assistance from the FDA came from testimony of Massachusetts pharmacy inspector Sam Penta.

97 **"Oh, it's nothing to be concerned about":** Dr. Ritu Bhambhani testified at Cadden's criminal trial and recounted these interactions, and her handwritten notes of her call with Cadden were included in the court's exhibits, which I obtained and used to confirm her memory of the interaction.

98 **He reassured Gieske:** Cadden's downplaying of the seriousness of his company's drug recall was the subject of Minnesota nurse Michelle Gieske's testimony at his trial, and was supported by her September 27, 2012, emails with Cadden and her colleagues.

98 **Owen Finnegan and Joe Connolly were gowned up:** Glenn Chin and Barry Cadden's orders to stop production and scour the clean room before the FDA and Massachusetts inspections were confirmed by multiple NECC employees, including Owen Finnegan and Joseph Connolly.

99 **Inside the spartan New England district office:** Scenes and conversations related to the FDA's inspection of NECC were derived from the testimony of the agency's pharmacy inspector, Stacey Degarmo, and microbiologist Almaris Alonso. Each also filed written reports, and some of their emails were obtained among the court exhibits.

105 **As they waited to reenter NECC, Degarmo's team:** This detail was alluded to in the FDA's reports, and confirmed by assistant U.S. attorney

George Varghese, the federal government's lead investigator who interviewed all of the FDA inspectors about NECC.

106 **The drugs, all from the August 10 lot:** Details of the rush to confirm fungus in NECC's confiscated drug vials was included in the FDA microbiologist Philip Istafanos's testimony in multiple federal criminal trials, as well as FDA emails, reports, and other criminal case exhibits.

CHAPTER 8. OCTOBER DELUGE

109 **Dr. Park spoke slowly:** This call was transcribed, and additional details were sourced from news coverage of the announcement and interviews with Dr. Benjamin Park and others at the CDC.

109 **The CDC estimated that 13,534 patients:** Dr. Rachel Smith et al., "Fungal Infections Associated with Contaminated Methylprednisolone Injections," *New England Journal of Medicine* 369 (2013): 1598–609.

111 **CDC opened up its Emergency Operations Center:** Details about the previous incidents during which the CDC opened its emergency operations center come from the agency's website. Additional scene details came from my visit to the facility and interviews with CDC staff.

111 **The call took Joyce Lovelace:** The scene of the St. Thomas pain clinic's call to Joyce Lovelace about her husband's case came from interviews with Joyce and her daughter, Karen Talbott, at the Lovelace home in Albany, Kentucky.

112 **Chin saw them watching:** This scene's details and those comprising the final hours at NECC came from interviews and the testimony of former employees, particularly Owen Finnegan, Annette Robinson, and Joseph Connolly.

113 **It wasn't until Connolly turned on the television:** Ibid.

113 **They were in Lyn's hospital room:** Details for this scene came from interviews with Penny Laperriere in Ann Arbor, Michigan, as well as emails she shared between her and the Channel 4 reporter, which confirmed the date and time.

114 **Next, she dialed Michigan Pain Specialists:** Details of this call came from interviews with Penny Laperriere and the testimony of Dr. Edward Washabaugh in Barry Cadden's trial.

114 **Dr. Varsha Moudgal learned the answer:** I put this scene together based on information from two interviews with Dr. Varsha Moudgal, and I

confirmed that the NPR story ran that day via the Internet Archive's Wayback Machine.

116 **Willard "J.R." Mazure:** Scenes and the details of Willard Mazure's case were reconstructed from interviews with him and his wife, Linda Mazure, at their home in Pinconning, Michigan. Willard also kept a journal of his hospital stay and took lots of photos with his cell phone, which he shared with me. His physician, Dr. Anurag Malani at St. Joseph Mercy Hospital in Ann Arbor, also confirmed certain clinical details with me.

118 **Down the way from Mazure's hospital room:** Details of Ray and Gayle Gipson's story came from multiple interviews with Ray at his home in Ypsilanti, Michigan, and Gayle's personal calendars and medical records, which he shared with me.

119 **Day 28, October 15, 2012; 15 dead, 214 cases:** Centers for Disease Control and Prevention outbreak update, October 15, 2012.

119 **The construction worker J.R. Mazure:** These case numbers were confirmed by St. Joseph Mercy Hospital infectious disease chiefs Dr. Varsha Moudgal and Dr. Anurag Malani, and by the CDC.

120 **The CDC assembled the world's foremost medical mycologists:** Dr. Tom Chiller at the CDC, an expert in fungal diseases who led the clinical team during the outbreak, helped assemble the Gang of Six medical mycologists: John Bennett of the National Institutes of Health, John Perfect of Duke University, Thomas Patterson of the University of Texas at San Antonio, Peter Pappas of the University of Alabama at Birmingham, Carol Kauffman of the University of Michigan, and Dimitrios Kontoyiannis of the University of Texas MD Anderson Cancer Center.

120 **The next was the nuclear option:** Information about the antifungal treatment options come from interviews with doctors. Other sources include Ana Espinel-Ingroff, "History of Medical Mycology in the United States," *Clinical Microbiology Reviews* 9, no. 2 (April 1996): 235–72; Matthew C. Fisher et al., "Worldwide Emergence of Resistance to Antifungal Drugs Challenges Human Health and Food Security," *Science* 360, no. 6390 (2018): 739–42.

121 **He was given 450 milligrams of "amphoterrible":** The initial doses given to fungal meningitis patients at St. Joe's were 5 to 7.5 mg/kg of amphotericin B and 6 mg/kg of voriconazole twice daily. J.R. Mazure weighed about 95 kilograms when he first got sick. J.R. confirmed his dosages via photographs he took of the drugs the hospital was giving him.

122 **Some underwent four or more spinal taps:** Information from St. Joseph Mercy Hospital and the testimony of Dr. Edward Washabaugh in the Cadden trial.

122 **When she burst into Lyn's room:** This hospital scene was built from multiple interviews with Penny Laperriere in Ann Arbor, Michigan, photos from her phone, and a visit to St. Joseph Mercy Hospital.

125 **There on Mazure's scan was a malignant-looking mass sitting in a bundle of his nerves:** Interview with St. Joe's radiologist, Dr. Spencer Koch, in his lab at St. Joseph Mercy Hospital, where he demonstrated how he read the MRI scans from the outbreak and detailed his work to identify the abscesses.

126 **One doctor thought to himself:** These details come from an interview with Dr. Spencer Koch at St. Joseph Mercy Hospital. Dr. Koch was among the first doctors to see and describe fungal abscesses in the crush of patients early in outbreak.

126 **An incredible 153 people had been diagnosed:** Patient data comes from Dr. Varsha Moudgal et al., "Spinal and Paraspinal Fungal Infections Associated with Contaminated Methylprednisolone Injections," *Open Forum Infectious Diseases* 2014 Mar; 1(1): ofu022, doi: 10.1093/ofid/ofu022.

126 **The fungus was pinkish:** Details from the operating room at St. Joe's came from the author's background interviews with surgeons at St. Joseph Mercy Hospital in Ann Arbor.

127 **Over the next six weeks:** Ibid.

128 **Now the team finally had the raw numbers:** Kainer's initial attack rate data for each lot of contaminated steroids—calculated in mid-October as hundreds around the country were diagnosed—would hold up. A CDC study after the outbreak reported: "On the basis of data from case-report forms received as of July 1, 2013, the lot-specific attack rates were estimated to be 6 cases per 1,000 ml of methylprednisolone acetate used from lot 05212012@68, 40 cases per 1,000 ml from lot 06292012@26, and 22 cases per 1,000 ml from lot 08102012@51." See Dr. Rachel Smith et al., "Fungal Infections Associated with Contaminated Methylprednisolone Injections," *New England Journal of Medicine* 369 (2013): 1598–609.

CHAPTER 9. AN OPPORTUNISTIC KILLER

131 **Bloodthirsty—that's how Dr. Ben Park described the fungus:** This characterization of the fungal pathogen *E. rostratum* came from my

interviews with Dr. Benjamin Park at CDC. Further research: Jana M. Ritter et al., "Exserohilum Infections Associated with Contaminated Steroid Injections," *American Journal of Pathology* 183, no. 3 (September 2013): 881–92.

131 **The first mention of the microbe:** Charles Drechsler, "Some Graminicolous Species of Helminthosporium," *Journal of Agricultural Research* 24, no. 8 (1923): 641–740.

132 **Of an estimated 1.5 to 5.1 million species of fungi:** Gregory M. Mueller and John Paul Schmit, "Fungal Biodiversity: What Do We Know? What Can We Predict?" *Biodiversity and Conservation* 16, no. 1 (January 2007): 1–5. See also: Meredith Blackwell, "The Fungi: 1, 2, 3 . . . 5.1 Million Species?" *American Journal of Botany* 98, no. 3. (March 2011): 426–38.

132 **Due to the work of Agostino Bassi:** J. R. Porter, "Agostino Bassi Bicentennial (1773–1973)," *Bacteriology Reviews* 37, no. 3 (September 1973): 284–88. See also "Agostino Bassi" in *Encyclopaedia Britannica.*

133 **At the turn of the twentieth century:** Ana Espinel-Ingroff, "History of Medical Mycology in the United States," *Clinical Microbiology Reviews* 9, no. 2 (April 1996): 235–72.

134 **Each night after dinner with his family:** Details of Charles Drechsler's life and physical appearance come from archival photographs at the Botany Libraries photograph collection, Harvard University. Also Robert D. Lumsden, "Charles Drechsler, 1892–1986," *Mycologia* 79, no. 3 (May–June 1987): 345–52.

136 **After Drechsler named his gnarled, scarred fungus:** K. J. Leonard and Edna G. Suggs, "*Setosphaeria prolata*, the Ascigerous State of *Exserohilum prolatum*," *Mycologia* 66, no. 2 (1974): 281–97. Further details were gleaned from an interview of Leonard by journalist Jennifer Frazer in *Scientific American*, published November 13, 2012, https://www .scientificamerican.com/article/fungal-meningitis-pathogen -discovers-new-appetite-human-brains.

137 **The invention of disposable, preloaded plastic syringes:** Charles E. Myers, "History of Sterile Compounding in U.S. Hospitals: Learning from the Tragic Lessons of the Past," *America Journal Health-System Pharmacy* 70, no. 16 (August 15, 2013).

138 **In 1926, the U.S. Pharmacopeia . . . for the first time listed two injectable medications:** Committee on National Formulary of the American Pharmaceutical Association, *The National Formulary*, 5th ed. (Washington, DC: American Pharmaceutical Association, 1926), 2–7.

138 **But at 37 degrees Celsius in a CDC lab:** The agency's tests in the early days of the outbreak were described and characterized in an interview by Dr. Tom Chiller, chief of CDC's Mycotic Diseases Branch.

138 **When a pathogen invades:** My simplistic descriptions of some of the body's immune system responses come from interviews with multiple doctors who are characters in this book, as well as from information in the book *An Elegant Defense: The Extraordinary New Science of the Immune System* by Matt Richtel (New York: HarperCollins, 2019). Information about the body's oxidative bursts comes from Adilia Warrisa and Elizabeth R. Ballou, "Oxidative Responses and Fungal Infection Biology," *Seminars in Cell & Developmental Biology* 89 (May 2019): 34–46.

CHAPTER 10. THE CASE OF A CAREER

141 **George Varghese typed "fungal meningitis":** The scenes of assistant U.S. attorney George Varghese learning about the case came from multiple interviews with him at his office in Boston, his co-counsel, and the paralegal that worked with him on the NECC case.

142 **Amanda Strachan stood in her office:** Assistant U.S. attorney Amanda Strachan's story came from interviews with her, her co-counsel at the U.S. Attorney's Office in Boston, and the paralegal who worked on the case.

144 **Yeager assigned Strachan to manage the discovery phase:** Details of Strachan's early role came from her and from her partner on the NECC case, George Varghese, and were confirmed by their paralegal.

146 **A lawyer hired by the NECC called Finnegan:** The Conigliaro family's hiring of lawyers to represent NECC employees with company-funded attorneys was a fact presented as evidence in both the Barry Cadden and Glenn Chin trials. Finnegan and others confirmed this in interviews and/or testimony.

CHAPTER 11. THE HAIL MARY

152 **Within days an email from an old colleague:** Email from the FDA shared with the author by Sarah Sellers.

152 **Day 58, November 14, 2012; 32 dead, more than 400 cases:** CDC case numbers taken from daily update, November 13, 2012.

152 **Joyce Lovelace faced the row:** All testimony from the House and Senate committee hearings on the outbreak were video-recorded by each

chamber of Congress, and transcripts are publicly available on government websites.

153 **These criticisms:** Details of the strategy undertaken by the lobbying group International Academy of Compounding Pharmacists, which recently changed its name to the American Association of Compounding Pharmacists, come from the agency's own newsletters at the time of the outbreak, an interview with one of its lobbyists working at the time, and a half-dozen congressional staffers from both parties who worked on the legislation.

154 **Congresswoman Blackburn accepted a $10,000 donation:** All campaign finance data comes from the Center for Responsive Politics's OpenSecrets database: https://www.opensecrets.org.

159 **"Everything didn't work":** Jennifer Boyer's information comes from interviews with her in Washington and by phone, emails obtained by the author, and interviews with her colleagues on the U.S. Senate HELP committee.

159 **The Senate's draft bill:** All versions of the two bills that took form in the House and Senate are available through the Congress.gov website.

160 **Day 286, July 1, 2013; 61 dead, 749 cases:** See Dr. Rachel Smith et al., "Fungal Infections Associated with Contaminated Methylprednisolone Injections," *New England Journal of Medicine* 369 (2013): 1598–609.

160 **Ten months had passed since Tom Rybinski arrived:** The CDC tracks cases in an outbreak from the beginning of it to the end of the outbreak. In the case of the NECC fungal meningitis outbreak, the final tally found: as of July 1, 2013, a total of 749 cases in twenty states, with 61 deaths. The U.S. Attorney's Office investigation would use insurance claims, medical records, and health care data collected during its investigations to update this figure in 2019 to 103 deaths and more than 800 cases. See Dr. Rachel Smith et al., "Fungal Infections Associated with Contaminated Methylprednisolone Injections," *New England Journal of Medicine* 369 (2013): 1598–609.

161 **David Miller took emergency action:** Details of the IACP's lobbying campaign came from the group's own materials, including newsletters obtained by the author, interviews with congressional staffers, campaign finance records, and an interview with one of the group's lobbyists at the time.

162 **Roberts's tough talk:** Details from Jennifer Boyer's perspective come from interviews with her, emails, and IACP records. See also "Drug

Companies Plan to Use Compounding Bill to Eliminate Competition," July 14, 2013, by Alliance for Natural Health.

163 If House Republicans would not agree: Details of the genesis of the voluntary compounding regulatory option in the Food, Drug, and Cosmetic Act—Section 503B—come from multiple HELP and House Energy and Commerce Committee staffers from both parties who worked on the bill, lobbyists for the pharmacy and hospital industries involved in the negotiations, and congressional records.

CHAPTER 12. DEPRAVED INDIFFERENCE

167 2014: 76 dead, 778 fungal infections: These updated numbers were compiled by the U.S. Attorney's Office after the CDC had stopped tracking the outbreak. They were delivered to U.S. attorney Eric Holder on November 24, 2014, as prosecutors sought his approval of the indictment investigation against the NECC defendants.

167 George Varghese picked up his camera: The scenes of Varghese and Strachan's investigative visit to NECC were built using photographs Varghese took, interviews with both of them, and descriptions of what they found written in case documents in the trials of Barry Cadden and Glenn Chin.

167 Investigators had seized some twenty million pages: This number comes from Clare Reidy, the U.S. attorney's lead paralegal on the case who helped organize the database of NECC documents seized in the investigation.

169 The soft-spoken, neatly dressed man: Details of Strachan's interview with Kenneth Todd came from interviews with her and Varghese, Strachan's personal calendars, a reporting trip to Ann Arbor, and her notes.

170 Emma Todd died in March 2013: Emma Todd was one of the twenty-five victims whose cases were used in the murder counts against both Barry Cadden and Glenn Chin. Details of her illness and final days came from trial testimony and interviews with federal prosecutors.

172 The plainclothes agents were indistinguishable: Details of the FBI's arrest of Glenn Chin at Boston Logan International Airport came from interviews with the federal prosecutors involved in the arrest, as well as court documents and public statements made by defense attorneys. Glenn

Chin's defense attorney, Stephen Weymouth, also contributed information from Chin's perspective.

173 **Varghese and Strachan arrived:** Scene details of the federal prosecutors' presentation to U.S. attorney general Eric Holder came from multiple interviews with George Varghese and Amanda Strachan, copies of the slide presentation they gave, their emails before and after, photos of the conference room where they presented, and the U.S. Department of Justice's historical materials about the artwork and interior design of the room.

176 **His lawyer, Bruce Singal:** Bruce Singal and Michelle Peirce declined multiple requests to be interviewed for this book, but did provide defense exhibits and helpful context for their defense case. All other biographical materials and quotes were sourced to transcripts of court proceedings, videos Bruce Singal made describing his philosophical approach to trial law, court documents, and audio and video of statements Singal made to the press.

CHAPTER 13. TRIAL

180 **Varghese's opening statement:** The scenes from Barry Cadden's trial were built from multiple sources. All direct quotations come from the trial transcripts. Any reactions to testimony, or thoughts or feelings of someone involved in the case, were either noted in the transcript or described by the person in interviews. The author also attended the trial in 2018 of NECC co-owner Greg Conigliaro, operations director Sharon Carter, and four of its pharmacists. Many of the witnesses called during that trial also testified against Cadden, so any physical descriptions of them came from firsthand reporting.

200 **In the deliberation room, juror Melanie Gomes:** The scene inside the deliberation room was built through multiple interviews by phone with juror Melanie Gomes, who was one of the key jurors who refused to vote for a guilty verdict for the murder counts against Barry Cadden. I also used information from three other jurors who did brief media interviews after the verdict.

EPILOGUE

207 **2019–2020: more than 100 dead, 793 cases:** These were the latest outbreak-related numbers compiled by the U.S. Attorney's Office in Boston.

207 **The boxy brick building:** From a reporting trip to NECC's former building in Framingham in September 2018 and November 2019.

209 In the Detroit suburb of New Hudson: Przydzial's story and case details came from interviews with him and Donna in Michigan, and his medical records.

213 In 2016, nurses in the pediatric units of hospitals: Details of the Pharmakon case came from legal documents I obtained through PACER, the federal courts online database, and a news release from the U.S. Attorney's Office when the case was filed.

214 An effort by the Pew Charitable Trusts: Pew began this effort under the guidance of Elizabeth Jungman, who left the Senate HELP Committee after passage of the DQSA and led Pew's efforts to study and publicize problems with the industry. She was an invaluable source while at Pew, which she left in 2019 to take a job at the FDA. Pew's spreadsheet of adverse events caused by compounding errors is available on the group's website.

214 In 2016, seventeen people in New York: Details of these two cases are published on CDC's website.

215 In 2017, during cataract surgeries and other procedures: Details of the Guardian case came from federal court documents, FDA records accessed through the FDAzilla website, and an excellent story about the case in BuzzFeed News: Stephanie M. Lee, "At Least 68 People Are Nearly Blind After a Botched Drug Was Injected into Their Eyeballs," BuzzFeed, September 21, 2018.

215 Medicare Part D spending: Government Accountability Office Report (GAO-17-64), "Drug Compounding-FDA Has Taken Steps to Implement Compounding Law, but Some States and Stakeholders Reported Challenges" (November 2016).

216 Meanwhile, hospitals: U.S. Department of Health and Human Services Office of Inspector General, "Most Hospitals Obtain Compounded Drugs from Outsourcing Facilities, Which Must Meet FDA Quality Standards" (June 2019): OEI-01-17-00090. Note: Despite the title of the report, it actually confirmed that a significant number of hospitals admitted to using non-FDA approved compounders—11 percent.

217 According to FDA records, some have been recently cited: I obtained a list from HHS via the Freedom of Information Act that had forty-five compounding pharmacies that the OIG determined were selling drugs to hospitals without FDA approval. I ran this list through the FDAzilla database to obtain warning letters and other records about each facility.

217 Republican congressman Morgan Griffith of Virginia: Copies of Representative Griffith's bills are available via the Congress.gov website.

INDEX

Page numbers in italics indicate photos.

AIDS, 136
Alexander, Lamar, 157–58, 161
Allen, Loyd, 79
Alliance for Pharmacy Compounding
    (formerly International Academy
    of Compounding Pharmacists
    [IACP]), 80, 83–84, 86, 153–55,
    158, 161–62, 217
Allred, Anna, 48–49
Alonso, Almaris, 101–5
American Pharmacists Association, 83
Ameridose, 20, 23–24, 153
amphotericin B, 120–21, 136
Analytical Research Laboratories,
    200–201
antifungal medications, 11,
    120–21, 136
Apophysomyces trapeziformis fungus, 42
Aspergillus fumigatus fungus
    culture photo, *5*
    nationwide alert regarding, 46
    testing for, 36, 39–40, 49, 128–29
attack rates, prioritizing treatment by,
    127–28
autopsies
    of Effie Elwina Shaw, 48–49
    requests from the CDC, 124–25

bacteria, 106, 108
Barton, Joe, 155

Bassi, Agostino, 132–33
Baxter, Karina, 202
Bearden, Caprice, 213–14
Benham, Rhoda, 133–34
Bhambhani, Ritu, 97
Big Pharma, 14, 17, 78
biological indicators, 65
biological warfare, 41
Blackburn, Marsha, 154–55
Blumenfeld, Michael, 31
Bond, Kit, 82–83
Boyer, Dave, 162
Boyer, Jennifer, 159, 162
Brandt, Mary, 129
Brent, Paula, 203
Brown, Dennis, 146–47
Brown, Rachel Fuller, 134, 135–36

Cadden, Barry
    arrest and criminal trial, 166,
        176–78, 179–80, 183–85, 190,
        196–99, 201–6
    backfilling names on large orders,
        28–29, 55
    "bulletproof" NECC drug testing
        policy, 55–57
    and CDC investigation of NECC,
        93–95
    concerns about NECC's liability, 37,
        112–13